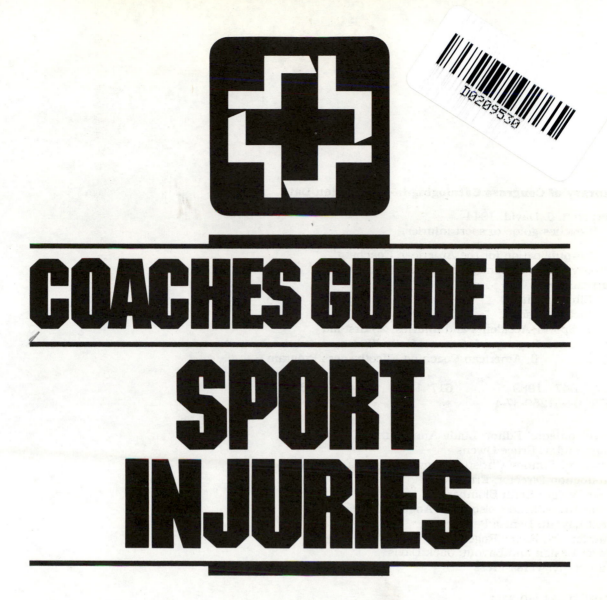

COACHES GUIDE TO SPORT INJURIES

A publication for the
American Coaching Effectiveness Program
Master Series (Level 2) Sport Science Curriculum

J. David Bergeron, MEd
Holly Wilson Greene, PhD, ATC, RPT

Indiana University
Library
Northwest

RD
97
.B47
1989

Sum

HUMAN KINETICS BOOKS
Champaign, Illinois

Library of Congress Cataloging-in-Publication Data

Bergeron, J. David, 1944-
   Coaches guide to sport injuries.

   "A publication for the American Coaching
Effectiveness Program, level 2 sport injuries
curriculum."
   Bibliography: p.
   Includes index.
   1. Sports--Accidents and injuries. 2. First aid
in illness and injury.   I. Greene, Holly Wilson,
1946-   . II. American Coaching Effectiveness Program.
III. Title.
RD97.B47   1989   617'.1027   88-13674
ISBN 0-931250-37-4

Developmental Editor: Linda Anne Bump, PhD
Copy Editor: Bruce Owens
Assistant Editors: Christine Drews and Julia Anderson
Production Director: Ernie Noa
Text Design: Keith Blomberg
Typesetters: Brad Colson and Angela Snyder
Text Layout: Denise Peters
Interior Art: Ranee Rogers
Cover Design and Layout: Jack Davis
Printed by: Versa Press

ISBN: 0-931250-37-4

Copyright © 1989 by J. David Bergeron and Holly Wilson Greene

Notice. It is not the intent of the authors or the publisher that this textbook be used as a standard of care for injured athletes and other persons. This book is meant to be a part of the user's formal training in sport injury prevention and care. The procedures presented in this text represent accepted practices in the United States. Some procedures may not be part of the standard of care in all localities. It is the reader's responsibility to have the certification required to render emergency care to injured athletes, to know and follow all local care protocols, and to stay informed of any emergency care procedure changes.

Forms on pages 6 and 8 may be reproduced for use in your program. Except for use in a review, the reproduction or utilization of any other portion of this work in any form or by any electronic, mechanical, or other means, now known or hereafter invented, including xerography, photocopying and recording, and in any information retrieval system, is forbidden without the written permission of the publisher.

Printed in the United States of America

10 9 8 7 6 5 4 3 2 1

Human Kinetics Books
A Division of Human Kinetics Publishers, Inc.
Box 5076, Champaign, IL 61825-5076
1-800-342-5457
1-800-334-3665 (in Illinois)

ACEP Master Series (Level 2) Sport Science Courses

ACEP Master Series (Level 2) sport science courses are available to accompany the following texts.

Coaches Guide to Sport Law by Gary Nygaard and Thomas H. Boone. The authors explain a coach's legal responsibilities in easy-to-understand terms and give practical advice for improving standards of care and safety for athletes.

Coaches Guide to Time Management by Charles Kozoll. This innovative text shows coaches how to improve their self-organization and how to avoid the harmful effects of stress by controlling the pressures inherent in many coaching programs.

Coaches Guide to Sport Physiology by Brian Sharkey leads coaches step-by-step through the development of fitness-training programs suitable for their sport and for the athletes they coach.

Coaches Guide to Sport Injuries by David Bergeron and Holly Wilson Greene gives coaches information on injury prevention and on the immediate treatment and follow-up care for common athletic injuries.

Coaches Guide to Teaching Sport Skills by Robert W. Christina and Daniel M. Corcos uses practical coaching examples to take coaches through the teaching/learning process and offers coaches valuable advice for improving their teaching effectiveness.

Coaches Guide to Sport Psychology by Rainer Martens presents information on motivation, communication, stress management, the use of mental imagery, and other fascinating topics for enhancing coach-athlete relationships and for stimulating improved sport performances.

Each course consists of a *Coaches Guide*, a *Study Guide*, and a *Workbook*. ACEP certification is awarded for successful course completion. For more information about these courses, contact:

ACEP
Box 5076
Champaign, IL 61825-5076
1-800-342-5457
1-800-334-3665 (in Illinois)

Acknowledgments

We would like to take this opportunity to thank those individuals at Human Kinetics and the American Coaching Effectiveness Program who helped, guided, and encouraged us throughout the development of this project. A very special thanks goes to Linda Anne Bump, PhD, who held the task of turning our manuscript into a book. Her advice, evaluations, and patience are greatly appreciated.

The approaches to the prevention of sport injuries, detection and assessment of those injuries, and the initial care rendered at the scene vary according to the level of training of the care provider and the state in which the care is given. We received help from a number of professionals concerning improved prevention and care procedures taking place recently in the United States. We would like to thank the following individuals for their reviews and suggestions:

Dr. Michael Charles
   Ortho-East, Berkeley, CA

Dr. Paul G. Dyment
   Chief of Pediatrics, Maine Medical Center, Portland, ME

Melinda Flegel
   St. Francis Medical Center, Peoria, IL

Dr. Charles E. Hutcheson, Jr.
   DDS, Rph, Midlothian, VA

Dr. Michael A. Nelson
   West Mesa Pediatric Associates, Albuquerque, NM

Dr. Paul M. Taylor
   Division of Orthopaedics, Georgetown University Hospital, Washington, DC

Contents

Introduction

Coaches hold the responsibility for the safety and care of their athletes. This is true even in systems where trainers carry out certain duties of care and rehabilitation. Regardless of who does the daily planning and who provides the hands-on care, the responsibility still lies with the coach.

Most coaches work in public school systems and recreational and park leagues. These individuals do not have specially trained personnel to help them ready playing surfaces, organize emergency care supplies, keep track of the health of each athlete, assess injuries, render emergency care, and guide the injured athletes through physician-approved rehabilitation programs. All of these duties fall on the coach and volunteers. In such a situation, it is obvious that the coach is responsible for the athletes' safety and care.

Even where someone else is responsible for rendering care, the coach should know as much as possible about athletic injuries, injury care, and rehabilitation. The more the coach knows about the types of injuries common to all sports, those specific to his or her own sport, and how these injuries occur (the mechanism of injury), the more likely it is that the coach will be able to prevent most major injuries. The prevention of injuries must be a primary goal of the coach. Special training in injury prevention, assessment, care, and rehabilitation will help the coach prevent injuries and minimize the pain and damage associated with them.

Coaches who are trained in sport injury prevention and care and emergency care procedures have increased awareness of how injury prevention is directly related to their attitude and that of athletes. Daily interaction with the athletes and specific sessions on safety allow coaches to teach their athletes the importance of a proper attitude toward sports and toward injury prevention.

This textbook and its study guide have been designed to introduce you to sport injuries, injury assessment, emergency care, and the process of rehabilitation. Not all injuries are covered in this text. Instead, the text is limited to common sport injuries and to life-threatening injuries that require basic life support. Should an unusual injury occur, the basic care guidelines in this text will allow the person providing care to prevent additional harm while waiting for professional help.

In order to assess and care for injuries, most localities require some form of certification. This certification may be limited to American Heart Association or American Red Cross basic life support. More likely, the required certification will be Red Cross First Aid and Emergency Care. In some states a specific program in sport medicine is available. You should seek the highest available level of certification and stay up-to-date with the procedures expected at your level of training. To accomplish this, you will need more than the academic training provided by a textbook; that is, you will need to participate in a first aid course recognized as meeting the standards set by your state or community.

PART I

Understanding Sport Injuries

Chapter 1
Sport Injuries— The Coach's Role

Participation in a sport is a special time in life for most people, and the joy it brings can be greatly reduced or quickly erased by injury. As a coach, you will have the responsibility to provide the safest possible experience for your athletes and ensure that any injured athlete receives prompt and efficient care.

THE NATURE OF SPORT INJURIES

Injuries in sport activities can occur for many reasons. No matter how safe the environment or how well conditioned the athlete, activity will inevitably produce some injuries, whether it be by contact with other bodies, the floor or ground, or sporting equipment. Situations that cause a temporary loss of body control may produce injuries ranging from minor to severe. Usually, though, these injuries are minor.

Most injuries can be prevented. When prevention is not made an integral part of the program, an increase in injuries and true emergencies results. For example, an athlete may have a preexisting condition that he or she is not aware of. This can lead the way to injury. Another athlete may not be properly or completely rehabilitated from an injury before returning to action and constantly suffers new sprains and strains and reinjures him- or herself before healing can take place. Or perhaps an athlete has not been taught the skills needed to participate, has not been properly conditioned during the preseason, or has been allowed to neglect conditioning during the season. This individual, too, may injure him- or herself as well as others.

The prevention of injuries is covered in detail in chapter 2. For now, consider the coach as the main line of defense against injuries. When the coach's role in regard to injury is defined and the coach meets those responsibilities that are part of his or her role, the number and severity of such injuries can be reduced.

ROLES AND RESPONSIBILITIES

The coach's role in the initial care of athletes who are injured or suddenly ill can vary greatly depending on the responsibilities of the coach and the size of his or her organization. You may be coaching in a situation in which certified athletic trainers have the authority to make decisions about injured athletes, render all care that does not require a physician, direct rehabilitation under the guidance of a physician, and inform you as to when the athlete can rejoin the activity. Although many organizations have noted that certified trainers are needed in athletics and have made recommendations for the participation of trainers in all sports activities, there are many occasions when no trainers are available. In such situations, you may render the care, but there may be others who condition the athlete and control the rehabilitation programs. Even when certain responsibilities are given to others, you may have the ultimate responsibility for all aspects of care.

As a coach, you may have to assume any or all of the following responsibilities:

- Make certain that all athletes have a preseason physical examination. This will reduce the number of emergencies you will face by screening out some of those individuals with medical or physical problems that put them at risk when participating and by limiting the participation of others (see chapter 2).

- Have all necessary consent forms signed by the athletes, their parents, or their legal guardians. Because this consent allows for care to be initiated promptly, the severity of many injuries may be reduced by preventing additional complications.
- Have the athletes properly conditioned for their level of participation. Many sport injuries can be prevented or reduced in severity when the athletes have been properly conditioned.
- Monitor the general health and physical fitness of the athletes.
- Supply the required, high-quality equipment and protective gear and make certain that it is safe to use. You should have what is needed, not only what is traditional.
- Make certain that all equipment is properly fitted.
- Make certain that all exercise, conditioning, practice, play, and rehabilitation facilities, equipment, and apparatus are safe to use.
- Provide adequate protection from harsh environmental conditions even if it involves changing practice time or cancelling practice.
- Instruct the athletes in safety, injury prevention, and the use and care of protective gear.
- Develop the skills necessary for athletes to participate safely at their level of competition.
- Possess the required level of injury care and prevention skills and know how to apply these skills to help reduce certain injuries and accidents.
- Develop and carry out an emergency plan.
- Provide a proper field setup that includes water, ice, and a first aid kit containing all the items needed to render initial care.
- Assess the needs of athletes and exclude them from participation when required.
- Develop rehabilitation programs with attending physicians.
- Perform the proper field assessments for injury and sudden illness.

- Provide initial emergency care to the level of your training.
- Interact with the Emergency Medical Services (EMS) system to ensure a proper response to the emergency. In your area this could be part of the fire department, rescue squad, or a private ambulance service.

THE LEGAL ASPECTS OF EMERGENCY CARE

This section serves only as a general guide to the legal considerations given to emergency care—it is not meant to serve as legal advice. Before the start of your season, make certain that you have signed all the necessary contracts and have completed all the forms required by your organization, agency, school, company, or institution. Have a written description of your responsibilities in regard to rendering initial care. In addition, make certain that the athletes or their guardians have completed all the required forms. If you have any questions about your responsibilities, liabilities, or protection, you should seek the advice of professional legal counsel.

For more information concerning the law as it applies to the coach, see the ACEP Level 2 Sport Law Course described in the front of this book and *Coaches Guide to Sport Law* (Nygaard & Boone, 1985).

Important Legal Concepts

There are specific aspects of the law that apply to the rendering of prehospital emergency care for the injured and the suddenly ill. You should have a general knowledge of these aspects and know how they apply specifically in your locality.

Duty to Act

The first term you should be familiar with is the *duty to act*. In the past, this was applied to paid professional care providers and defined when they were required to provide care. Today, volunteer care providers have had their duty to act defined in many states. However, it is unclear what the coach's duty to act is when he or she has some training in providing emergency care.

As a coach, you have probably agreed to provide initial care in the event that an athlete is injured or becomes suddenly ill, and your athletes or their guardians have probably been made aware of this commitment. It is very likely that a court would consider you to have a duty to provide initial care when an athlete who is practicing, conditioning, competing, or rehabilitating is injured or becomes ill.

Standard of Care

The next concept is *standard of care*. Each state has established laws that indicate that, when emergency care is rendered, it must be provided within certain guidelines and to a given level of quality. The standard of care is usually based on state laws and the guidelines published by government agencies, EMS systems, and emergency care organizations and societies. Each person who provides care can be judged in terms of the care given relative to what others at the same level of training and experience would be able to do under the same circumstances.

The main problem with the standard of care for coaches who are providing initial care is that most states have very few specific laws and guidelines. The development of standards of care has focused mainly on the physician, nurse, allied health worker, and emergency medical technician (EMT). Some states do recognize guidelines set forth by boards of education, workshop courses, academic institutions providing sports medicine courses, and professional societies involved with injury in sports. The degree to which recognition has been given to these sources varies greatly. You will need to find out whether your state has laws or guidelines regarding a standard of care for coaches, including the specific procedures that are expected for given situations as well as the training that is required.

Since the standard of care for coaches may not be clearly defined in your state, certain state and national certifications can be important. For example, the American Heart Association (AHA) and the American Red Cross (ARC) both provide certification in basic life support, including clearing airway obstructions, rescue breathing, and performing cardiopul-

monary resuscitation, or CPR. If an athlete needs such care and if you are certified and provide the care you have been taught to provide, then you have provided the standard of care. Keep in mind that recertification is essential.

If you are certified in first aid and emergency care by the ARC and you provide the care that is required according to their guidelines, then you have met the standard of care. A problem would arise if you (a) failed to recognize or properly treat an injury according to standard ARC guidelines, (b) provided care using a technique that was not recognized by the ARC, or (c) applied a procedure that was beyond your level of training. Such actions might be proof of failing to provide the standard of care.

As you receive additional training, the standard of care that you are required to provide is upgraded. A problem may exist when you take any course work or study programs in sports medicine or receive a higher level of training in emergency care (e.g., as a First Responder or EMT). Although your only current ARC certification may be for a previous first aid course, the court may say that your additional knowledge of sport-injury care should have been applied in a given situation. This has yet to be tested in most localities. The standard recommendation is to do only what you have been trained to do and what is accepted by your state.

Much of the confusion about the standard of care as it relates to coaches providing initial care has been dealt with by having the coach follow the guidelines set forth by a medical board or medical director within his or her organization, school, or company. The coach who works in such a system is expected to provide the standard of care that this physician or group of physicians has formulated. Traditionally, the courts would hold the medical professionals responsible if they required you to do something that was not the correct standard of care. Today, in some areas, courts are questioning whether the coach is fully free of the responsibility to provide the correct standard of care when given an incorrect guideline. How this view applies to your locality will have to be answered by legal counsel.

It is important that you do only what you have been trained to do and that you keep a written record of the care you deliver. We

INJURY REPORT

Name _____   Date of Injury _____
             first   last

Address _____   Time of Injury _____

Phone _____   Location _____

I.D. No. _____   Sport _____

Classification: PE   IM   ATH   REC

Body Part Affected: (check)

Head	_____	Arm	_____	Thigh	_____
Neck	_____	Elbow	_____	Knee	_____
Shoulder	_____	Wrist	_____	Lower leg	_____
Back	_____	Hand	_____	Ankle	_____
Chest	_____	Finger	_____	Foot	_____
Hip	_____	Other	_____		

Nature of Injury: (check)

Severe cut	_____	Fracture	_____
Bruise	_____	Dislocation	_____
Strain	_____	Reinjury	_____
Sprain	_____	Other	_____

Describe How Injury Occurred: Signs and Symptoms:

_____   _____

_____   _____

Disposition: First aid rendered:

Released _____

Student health _____   Supplies Checked Out: (number)

Family physician _____   Elastic bandages _____

Hospital _____   Crutches _____

_____   Other _____
         Name of individual making report

_____   Returned _____ Date_____
Signature   Date

Witnesses:

(1) _____   (2) _____
Name

(1) _____   (2) _____
Address

(1) _____   (2) _____
Phone

PHYSICIAN'S REPORT

Diagnosis: Recommendations:

Disposition: Restrictions:

No practice until _____   Prescription:
                    date

Expected return to competition _____
                           date

Return appointment _____
                   date

_____
Signature   Date

recommend using an injury report form like the one on page 6 as a means to record all injuries and the care provided.

Negligence

The primary legal concern of individuals rendering emergency care is *negligence*. To the layperson, negligence usually implies that someone did not do what was expected or that what he or she did do was inappropriate. From a legal viewpoint, negligence is far more complicated. For negligence to be established, the following points must be met:

- The person providing the care must have a duty to act. This may be established since, as a coach, you assumed certain responsibilities for the athlete's care.
- The care that was provided did not meet the standard of care. Again, this may be a difficult point for the coach to define and understand unless there is a specific standard that is known and accepted by all the parties involved.
- The athlete must have been injured physically and/or emotionally by the care that was provided.

A legal professional would state that if these three points were made, negligence has yet to be established until some value is placed on the damage, at which time the provider would be required to give the victim money or some other form of compensation.

The three criteria imply potential problems for a coach who is providing initial emergency care; however, these problems have not gone unnoticed in many states. In an effort to help the providers of initial care and to ensure that care will be rendered without fear, many (but not all) states have laws to protect citizens when they attempt to help the sick and injured. These are the *Good Samaritan laws*. They have been developed to provide a certain amount of immunity from civil liability to individuals who provide initial emergency care. The laws require that the provider, to the best of his or her ability, act in good faith to render care to his or her level of training.

The Good Samaritan laws have become more complicated in the past 10 years. Some now exclude certain persons. For example, an EMT may be protected if this person is a volunteer but not when paid to be an EMT. There is a possibility that a paid coach who has assumed responsibility for initial care may not be protected unless a very specific standard of care has been established and followed. You will have to investigate the Good Samaritan laws in your state and follow the advice of legal counsel for your locality.

Consent

Any person who is receiving care has certain rights. A rational, aware adult is allowed by law to refuse care. This is true even when the adult has previously signed a form that allows for care to be delivered. The adult can simply say no to your offer to provide care. In fact, the adult does not have to say anything. If you try to provide care, and this person shakes his or her head to indicate "no," holds up a hand to indicate "stop," or pulls away from you, then an implied refusal of care must be recognized.

You must accept the fact that the adult athlete does not have to give you a reason why he or she has refused care. In addition, the reason given does not have to make sense to you. The person refuses your offer to help usually because of fear. The approach you should take is to establish the person's confidence through calm, quiet conversation.

If you attempt to provide care to an adult who is conscious and who has refused your care, you may find yourself facing charges of assault, battery, or the violation of civil rights. In the case of a refusal of care, you should have adult witnesses to your offer to help, to your explanations, and to the refusal. Be sure to note the witnesses' names and addresses. When possible, have the injured person sign a refusal-of-care form.

When you believe that an EMS response is required and the person has refused your care, you should still call for medical assistance because (a) the person may change his or her mind in a few minutes and strongly desire care; (b) the person may suffer a loss of consciousness that allows certain care procedures to be started; and (c) the arrival of trained professionals at the scene may help the athlete decide to accept care.

Actual Consent

When an adult signs a form allowing you to render care, should it be needed, or when an alert adult orally states that you can provide care, you have received *actual consent*. It is always best that the adult sign a consent form for the specific incident in which care is provided, but this is not practical in many cases. Even when you have a previously signed form of consent, make certain that you ask the person if you may help.

The actual consent for the care of a minor[1] can be granted by a parent or legal guardian prior to or during an emergency situation and is usually accomplished by having a parent or legal guardian sign a preconsent form prior to the start of the season (see below). When actual consent is given, care is to be provided even if the minor refuses care. However, this can create a problem since you cannot force care on anyone. You may have to gain the athlete's confidence before care can be provided. You should let the athlete know that the parents or guardians have consented to your providing any needed initial care.

Informed Consent

Actual consent is valid only if it is *informed consent*. The laws of informed consent are designed to cover the interactions between physicians and patients, especially when surgery is involved. At the coach's level, informed consent usually means that the athlete and/or guardian knows your training, what you believe is wrong, and what must be done.

Minor's Consent

If there is no previously signed consent form and the parents or guardians cannot be asked

---

[1]Always make certain that someone you believe to be a minor is actually a minor according to the laws of your state. The guidelines for defining a minor should be established prior to the season.

to give consent, *minor's consent* may apply to allow care to be given. This does not mean that the consent is given by the minor, but rather, minor's consent is a legal position that states that the parents or guardians would probably want care rendered if the minor had a life-threatening emergency or an injury that would cause very severe problems if it went untreated. Some states do not have minor's consent but still allow for the same course of action under the laws of implied consent.

Implied Consent

When an adult who has not signed a preconsent form is unconscious or is too sick or injured to give actual consent, then *implied consent* can be used to allow care to be started. Implied consent assumes that the individual would request help if he or she were able to do so. Implied consent is applied also to minors, the mentally ill, and developmentally disabled individuals (e.g., the mentally retarded) when legal guardians are not available to give consent and there is no preconsent form.

THE EMERGENCY PLAN

You should have a predetermined plan that allows for the proper assessment and care of athletes who have suffered injury or sudden illness. This plan should be developed and ready for use before the season begins and should be evaluated frequently so that refinements can be made. Whenever it is practical and appropriate, the plan should receive the input of your local EMS system, area emergency departments, team or attending physicians, school or company nurses, trainers,

---

Preconsent Form

I hereby give my permission for _____ to participate in _____.
Further, I authorize the school to seek emergency medical treatment for my child in the event of illness or injury if I cannot be contacted prior to treatment.

Date _____ Parent or Guardian _____

Address _____ Phone Number _____

Date _____ Parent or Guardian _____

Address _____ Phone Number _____

company safety officers, other coaches and staff, legal consultants, administrators, and the athletes.

Delegating Responsibility

An effective emergency plan requires the coach to delegate responsibilities. In some cases, it is possible to give certain responsibilities to mature adolescents, but whenever possible, they should be given to adults. Do *not* delegate essential tasks to children.

Your emergency plan should ensure that certain requirements are met. There must be someone who is responsible for alerting the EMS system when help is needed. This person must know the phone number of the EMS dispatch and the area poison-control center. You are responsible for having this person know where the nearest phone is located, the exact location of the sporting event, and what entrance can be used by the arriving EMTs.

Your emergency plan must cover whether access to the area of play is prevented by locked gates or doors. If so, you must have the necessary keys and assign someone to unlock these gates and doors.

An emergency plan must ensure that all necessary supplies and required personnel are on hand and organized for use. Also make sure that someone is assigned to bring the supplies to you when care must be provided and that persons who know how to assist you in moving the injured athlete are available.

Noting Phone Numbers

As part of your emergency plan, you must make certain that you have a list of all required phone numbers, including the EMS dispatch, local hospital emergency department, poison-control center, team physician, and local police department. If you are coaching a school team, you will probably need to include the phone numbers of the school health center, athletic director, and school principal. If you are a coach for a specific organization, company, or institution, then other phone numbers may be required.

Keep the list of required phone numbers in your first aid kit. You should also have the appropriate coins taped to the inside of this kit if the nearest telephone is a pay phone.

Whenever emergency care is given to an injured athlete, there should be someone assigned to record information while you render care. If the team does not have a trainer or if the trainer is not at the event, then you should carry a card file that contains the following information about each athlete, coach, assistant, and trainer:

- Name, address, telephone number, and age
- Name, address, and telephone number of the next of kin or legal guardian
- Religion (if pertinent)
- Name and phone number of the team physician and the athlete's family physician
- Names and phone numbers of any attending physicians, including those who are involved with rehabilitation programs
- Information on medical problems and allergies
- A record of injuries and the care provided
- The at-rest pulse and breathing rates

If the team has a trainer, this person would be responsible for developing and carrying the required card file. It is essential that these records be properly secured so that no one but you and the trainer have access to them. Otherwise, confidentiality may be lost.

You should have a responsible adult assigned to contact relatives or guardians and any physicians who may be needed for a particular incident. If this will be done after care has been rendered, then it is best if you place the calls.

Calling for Assistance

You must train the person who is going to place the call for an EMS response or contact other health care professionals. This person should know that it is necessary to relay his or her name, location, and the number from which he or she is calling. The person should be prepared to give the exact location of the incident, tell what has happened, how many people need help, their names and ages, and what is presently being done to help the injured or sick athletes. Tell this person that he or she should wait until the emergency dispatcher hangs up before disconnecting the call. This assures that the EMS dispatcher has all the required information.

Your emergency plan should always consider prevention as the first course of action. The elements of injury and illness prevention are discussed in chapter 2.

THE FIELD SETUP

All areas used by the athletes and any equipment, gear, or supplies should be checked prior to use. This procedure is discussed in chapter 2. The preactivity checklist must include all those items needed for the rendering of emergency care.

For each practice and event you should have water, ice packs, towels, and blankets. Store water in a cooler or in plastic squirt bottles.

Your supplies for care should include the following:

- Upper- and lower-extremity padded splint sets
- Triangular bandages for slings and swathes
- Cravats (cloth strips) for bandaging and for applying splints
- Sterile gauze pads, sterile bulky dressings, sterile occlusive dressings, self-adherent gauze roller bandages, plastic bandage strips (bandaids), and several rolls of 1½-inch athletic tape (may be split to various thicknesses to use as bandaging that will secure dressings)
- Tape adherent (liquid or aerosol spray)
- Elastic bandages (cotton), including at least one each in widths of 3, 4, and 6 inches (If there is room, pack two 4-inch-wide bandages.)
- Underwrap (one roll)
- Bandage shears and a tape cutter
- Tape remover
- Safety pins
- Nail clippers
- Tweezers
- Penlight flashlight
- Skin lubricant
- Antiseptic cleansing agent (e.g., 3% hydrogen peroxide)

- Antiseptic cream and/or solution
- Mild soap
- Mild analgesic balm (optional)
- Adhesive felt, vinyl foam, and moleskin
- Solution for wetting and cleaning hard and soft contact lenses
- Mirror
- Cotton swabs
- Tongue depressors

Select those items that will need to be carried to the athlete for true emergencies and place them in a well-labeled box, fishing tackle box, or suitable military or travel pack. Make certain that any splints are kept with this box or pack.

SUMMARY AND RECOMMENDATIONS

The actions taken by a coach can prevent many injuries and may reduce the severity of other injuries. These actions are part of the responsibilities of coaching and require the coach to follow specific guidelines that will ensure safe participation and, when necessary, the delivery of the standard of care for injured athletes. The coach must know and be able to follow these guidelines.

As you continue to study sport injuries, consider the following:

1. Follow the guidelines that apply to such matters as the health of the athlete, conditioning, skills training, rehabilitation, equipment, and a safe playing environment to help prevent most injuries.

2. For each injury studied, consider how your emergency plan, the supplies and personnel you will have available, and your own skill in providing initial emergency care can be utilized to provide the standard of care if one of your athletes sustains this specific injury.

3. Remember that the role of the coach continues beyond initial care. You will be expected to be involved in rehabilitating the athlete. When an injury occurs, one of your goals must be the athlete's safe return to participation.

Chapter 2
The Prevention of Sport Injuries

Where there is vigorous activity, there will always be injuries. However, these injuries should be minor—limited to small bruises, scrapes, minor muscle strains (pulls), and minor sprains—and easily cared for with basic first aid skills, rest, and basic rehabilitation exercises. Adequate preventive measures attempt to reduce minor injuries and eliminate the more serious ones that have been related to sport activities.

ELEMENTS OF PREVENTION

The elements of a good sport injury prevention program include the following:

- Medical support
- The athlete's attitude
- A safe environment
- Protective equipment
- Physical conditioning

Medical Support

A preseason physical should be required of all athletes regardless of age and past health record. Although this examination may disqualify some individuals, its main purpose is to detect potential problems that need to be considered by the physician, athlete, parents and guardians, and coaches. Most of the problems detected will not disqualify the athlete. But when disqualification does occur, a positive outcome is possible as the information gained often can be used to direct the athlete into a more appropriate sport.

The preseason physical should be one that will

- disqualify individuals who have abnormalities that place them at too high a risk to participate in certain contact sports; for example, those having only one eye, kidney, or testicle;
- disqualify individuals who have preexisting conditions that would place them at risk; for example, such conditions as certain cardiovascular, respiratory, renal (kidney), digestive (including the liver and pancreas), neurological (brain and nerve), musculoskeletal, and metabolic diseases (e.g., severe diabetes) (The nature of the problem and how it is controlled will require that decisions be made on an individual basis.);
- disqualify individuals with preexisting or recent injuries who would be at risk; for example, someone who has had a recent severe head injury, a history of concussions, a fracture that is not fully healed, a lax joint due to a previous severe sprain, and so on;
- point out those individuals who may need to have limited participation—for example, the athlete who is still recovering from injuries; someone with asthma, diabetes, high or low blood pressure, a convulsive disorder, heart disease, or a musculoskeletal disorder; or someone with a psychological or emotional disorder;
- point out those individuals who should be limited to instructional (noncompetitive) participation; for example, those who may have heart problems, limited vision, developmental disorders, or a number of

other factors that would prevent competitive participation or required aspects of training;

- point out individuals who need special attention; for example, an athlete who is over- or underweight, who is limited in flexibility (range of motion), or who needs specific physical development such as strengthening a weak ankle; and
- meet all legal and insurance obligations.

The ideal physical examination should include a history of immunizations, a reevaluation of past problems, and an evaluation of current problems. The physical work-up should include evaluations of weight, growth and development, blood pressure, heart, lungs, skin, head (including an eye test), oral cavity (including a dental exam for some sports), neck, trunk, groin, and extremities. Tests for flexibility, joint laxity, strength, and balance should be given. A urinalysis is recommended by some authorities, but the current trend is away from including laboratory tests in the preseason physical. Which aspects will be included in the physicals depend on local policies.

The coach should receive written notification of any problems that need special consideration or possible emergency care. This notification must be kept as a permanent record. An example of a preparticipation physical examination form is shown on page 13.

The role of physicians, including the team physician, should not be limited to the preseason physical. Their role in the assessment and care of injured athletes is obvious; however, their assistance in rehabilitation is often overlooked. You should contact the injured athlete's attending physician and obtain instructions for rehabilitation. The physician should be able to customize the program for the athlete and bring you up to date on new rehabilitation programs. Decisions to move an athlete from one level of rehabilitation to the next also may have to be made by the physician. Approval must be given by the attending physician before the athlete can return to participation.

Remember that physicians are not the only health care professionals that you may be dealing with. Before the start of the season, it is a good idea to meet with your local EMS squad or participating private ambulance company. If a school health official will be involved with

initial or follow-up care, then a preseason meeting should be scheduled with that individual as well. You need to discuss their roles, how to call for assistance, what they expect you to do, the most likely injuries, and any new procedures in basic cardiac life support (mouth-to-mouth rescue breathing, cardiopulmonary resuscitation [CPR], and so on). In addition, if your athletes will be sent to a physical therapy office or sports medicine clinic for rehabilitation, you need to meet with the therapist in charge of these programs to define your role during therapy.

As a coach, you should make every effort to allow those individuals who cannot participate in physical activities to be part of your program. As you define your needs during preseason planning, include training, managing, and assistant roles that can be filled by someone who is limited in participation but who still wants to be involved with the sport.

The Athletes' Attitude

It is the coach's responsibility to develop the athletes' attitude toward injury prevention, which requires that you tell them that you are serious about injury prevention. You should explain which types of injuries are common to the sport and how prevention can reduce their occurrence. Next, you need to warn the athletes of the more serious injuries that are possible and the steps you have taken to prevent them. At this point, you must emphasize how all these preventive measures depend on the athletes' cooperation. Prevention does not work unless the athletes realize that it is part of the sport and requires their involvement.

The athletes must be instructed to look out for the safety of themselves and of others. For example, the *privilege* of swinging a bat comes with the *responsibility* of making certain that it is safe to do so; and the *privilege* of being on the baseball team comes with the *responsibility* of staying alert for bats being swung and balls being hit and thrown. You must tell the athletes that if they wish to participate, a certain level of awareness must be maintained during practice and competition.

Athletes who are on the sidelines or waiting to participate are subject to injuries related to the activity or to improper behavior. You must emphasize that you consider these athletes to

ILLINOIS HIGH SCHOOL ASSOCIATION
PHYSICIAN'S CERTIFICATE
(PRINTED 1986-87)

No. _____

KEY
0 NO DEFECT
✓ SLIGHT DEFECT
X MARKED DEFECT

IF STUDENT TRANSFERS, THIS CARD SHOULD BE SENT TO THE NEW SCHOOL

NAME

ADDRESS

BIRTH DATE

REQUIRED:	YEAR	19	19	19	19	19	19
MONTH—DAY							
HEIGHT							
WEIGHT							
GEN. POSTURE							
HEART: Murmur							
Rhythm							
Blood Pres.							
RATE: Normal							
After 15 Hops							
After 2 Min.							
HERNIA							
LUNGS: Percussion							
Auscultation							
ORTHOPEDIC: Feet							
Spine							
CONTAGION:							

RECOMMENDED:	YEAR	19	19	19	19	19	19
URINE: Spec. Grav.							
Albumen							
Sugar							
Casts							
TONSILS							
NOSE AND THROAT							
GLANDS							
EARS: Right							
Left							
TEETH							
EYES: Right							
Left							
BLOOD TESTS:							
TUBERCULIN TEST:							
OTHER DEFECTS:							

IN THE SPACE BELOW, INDICATE ATHLETIC ACTIVITIES IN WHICH STUDENT SHOULD NOT PARTICIPATE:

EXAM. BY:

19___:_____ 1ST:_____ M.D. Date:_____
19___:_____ 2ND:_____ M.D. Date:_____
19___:_____ 3RD:_____ M.D. Date:_____
19___:_____ 4TH:_____ M.D. Date:_____
19___:_____ 5TH:_____ M.D. Date:_____

NOTE: COMMENT ON BACK OF CARD ON ANY DEFECT WHICH MIGHT BE HELPED THROUGH CORRECTIVE TREATMENT

Note. Reprinted courtesy of the Illinois High School Association.

be part of the game and expect them to stay aware of what is happening—they should stay "in the game." Some athletes who are on the sideline take a view of their position as "riding the bench." Boredom or attention seeking may lead to horseplay that could result in injury. You must not lose track of where these athletes are and what they are doing, and you must be sure that they feel they are a part of the activity, behave properly, and stay alert.

Your athletes are more likely to be serious about the prevention of injuries if they know how serious you are about the subject. Detail your respective roles in injury prevention, address injury prevention more than just at the beginning of the season, and set up rules to help reduce injuries.

Once you have established the rules, enforce them in a consistent manner. Let the athletes know that there are specific punishments for failing to obey the rules. But remember, punishments that involve physical activity, such as running laps, often produce negative results.

Finally, talk to the athletes about the reasons for their participation in the sport. Use this opportunity to discuss the dangers of playing injured or giving up personal safety to make a play, especially the physical dangers for the young, growing athlete. Too many children enter sports believing that they should crash into a wall or pole to make a play or that they should continue to run no matter how sore their leg may be. The reasons for participating and the limits of what can be safely done in practice and competition may be clouded by peer pressure or the misguidance of others. As a coach, you must establish the goals of the activity and how they relate to the prevention of injury.

A Safe Environment

It is the coach's responsibility to make certain that all playing surfaces, pools, and sporting equipment are safe for practice and participation. This rule holds true for both home and away games. For example, all equipment stored on sidelines should be far enough from the boundary lines to make a collision improbable. Wall mounted devices should be padded, and all lights should be protected to prevent glass from falling on participants if a bulb is broken.

All facilities should be free of debris and clean enough to comply with standards of good sanitation. Playing surfaces should be made of the correct materials and be of the correct consistency. A playing field with uncut grass or unfilled holes is not a safe surface. A track in disrepair should not be used by your athletes, nor should a dirty or poorly illuminated gymnasium, locker room, training room, shower, lavatory, or pool.

All the equipment and apparatus that is used should be of acceptable quality, in a good state of repair, and properly cleaned before use. You must inspect all equipment and apparatus and immediately remove or take out of service any item that does not pass inspection. Do not delay doing this since an unsupervised athlete may begin to use the equipment or apparatus while you are away from the scene.

The coach is also responsible for the athletes' exposure to excessive heat, cold, sun, smog and air pollution, and harsh environmental conditions. The specifics on these problems and preventive measures are discussed in chapter 13.

Protective Equipment

When a hazard cannot be eliminated, protective equipment is needed to decrease the chances or severity of injury. The effectiveness of equipment is greatly reduced if it is of poor quality, improperly fitted, or in a state of disrepair. Even if you have an equipment manager, the ultimate responsibility for the quality of protective equipment is yours.

You can avoid many of the problems associated with protective equipment by purchasing equipment only from authorized dealers. Before making any decisions, discuss your specific needs with representatives from various manufacturers. Seek the assistance of an experienced coach, athletic director, trainer, or team physician. Take into account the size, strength, and skill level of each athlete before ordering and assigning equipment.

In certain sports, there is a reluctance on the part of some coaches to require all the protective equipment that is needed. For example, there are ice hockey coaches who believe that protective headgear is an optional piece of equipment. This approach is hard to justify since studies have shown the importance of such protection, especially for the child athlete. Another example is found in women's lacrosse, where some coaches have stated that the rules of play eliminate the need for face protection and headgear. Obviously, the rules cannot prevent an errant ball from striking the head or face or a stick from being wielded by an undisciplined player. You should use logic, not tradition, to make protective-equipment decisions. If there is the chance of injury and if protective gear is manufactured, use the protective gear.

Unfortunately, there are times when the proper protective equipment is available but is not worn. You must discuss the equipment and its use with your athletes. Be sure to review the importance of each piece of protective equipment and why it must be properly fitted and kept in good order. Show your athletes how to use and care for the equipment and how to make quick inspections for defects or wear before and after each use.

Be sure to set up specific rules concerning equipment and have specific penalties for failing to obey the rules. Present these to the athletes and *always* enforce the rules; understand that these rules will vary depending on the sport, the optional equipment used along with the standard protective equipment, the individual responsible for cleaning and maintenance, and so on. Remember, however, that the penalties for rule infractions should *not* be physical activity. Some examples of the rules you may develop include the following:

- Protective equipment must be worn at all times during practice and competition.
- Protective equipment must not be modified or changed in any way without the consent of the coach, trainer, or team physician. In approving a modification, be sure that the change is safe. You may want to seek the advice of those who are more knowledgeable, including the manufacturer or its sales representative.
- Protective equipment must be properly used and never abused.
- All protective equipment must be properly fitted. Follow the manufacturer's recommendations for fitting. If you have any doubts, check with the manufacturer or its sales representative.

- Protective equipment must be properly cleaned and maintained. The athlete must check for defects and excessive wear immediately before and after using the equipment. Any defects must be reported immediately to the coach or equipment manager. All athletes must be instructed in how to examine their protective equipment for defects and excessive wear. Also, check with the manufacturer or sales representative for recommendations about cleaning and maintenance. Keep in mind that the wrong cleaning substance may reduce the protective quality of the equipment.
- No one is allowed to use damaged, defective, or excessively worn equipment.

Most coaches are familiar with the protective-equipment demands of their particular sport. Table 2.1 lists the basic protective-equipment needs for some popular sports. Notice that athletic shoes, protective eyewear and mouth guards are used in almost every sport. These items will be discussed in greater detail.

Athletic Shoes

You should convince your athletes to select their athletic shoes on the basis of sound reasoning rather than on fashion or "star" endorsement. Give them important pointers on selecting shoes, emphasizing that they should buy the highest quality that is affordable. During sport activity, the stresses placed on the feet demand more than the minimal support offered by cheap shoes, especially when the athlete's feet are still growing.

Let your athletes know that wearing the correct kind of shoe with a proper fit will minimize injury. For example, in football there is a noticeable decrease in ankle and knee injuries when soccer shoes are worn instead of the conventional cleats. For basketball, high-top shoes provide additional support for the unstable ankle. Shoes for basketball and racquet sports should be reinforced along the forefoot. This provides more support and protection for the foot and prolongs the life of the shoe. Young competitors in baseball should wear "tennis" shoes, running shoes, soccer shoes, all-turf shoes, or rubber-soled spikes, all of which decrease the likelihood of catching the foot during a slide or "spiking" a baseman while sliding.

Table 2.1
Protective Equipment—Basic Needs

Sport	Protective equipment
Badminton	Court shoes
Baseball/softball	Baseball gloves, baseball or soccer shoes or shoes with appropriate spikes for the skill level, batting helmets with ear protectors, long socks, long pants, sliding pads, athletic supporter for male athlete; for catcher: chest protector, shin guards, face mask with neck (throat) protector, cup supporter for male athlete
Basketball	High-top basketball shoes, knee pads, mouth guard, eyeglasses guard, athletic supporter for male athlete
Field hockey	Shin guards, long socks, mouth guard; for goalie: helmet with face mask, padded gloves, leg pads, and kickers
Football	Soccer shoes, knee pads, hip pads, thigh pads, shoulder pads, helmet with face mask, mouth guard, tight pants and jersey, cup supporter for male athlete
Gymnastics	Gymnastics slippers, hand grips, hip pads (when appropriate)
Handball	Court shoes, eye protector, padded gloves
Jogging/running	Training shoes, socks
Roller skating	Heavy socks, knee pads, elbow pads, helmet, gloves
Soccer	Soccer shoes, shin guards, long socks, athletic supporter for male athlete; for goalie: gloves
Swimming	Goggles
Tennis/racquetball	Court shoes, eye protector, glove
Volleyball	Court shoes, knee pads, long-sleeved jersey, athletic supporter for male athlete
Wrestling	Wrestling shoes, knee pads, elbow pads, headgear, mouth guard, athletic supporter for male athlete

Recently, the number of running shoes on the market has increased to the point where complete comparison shopping is impractical. You should direct your athletes to the better affordable brands that have proven to be both functional and reliable in the past. All running shoes, especially those designed for training, sacrifice support as more cushion is added to the midsole. Shoes with waffle, or ribbed, soles are designed for straightforward movement, traction, and shock absorption. They should not be worn for sports that require rapid, unpredictable changes in direction.

Direct your athletes to consider the following features when selecting shoes (see Figure 2.1):

- The support and snugness offered by the heel counter
- The fit and firmness of the arch support
- The thickness and flexibility of the sole, especially in the forefoot
- Stiffer soles if the shoes are going to be used on a hard surface

- Level heels that do not tilt inward or outward when the shoes are placed on a flat table

Fitting Athletic Shoes. Athletic shoes should fit comfortably and provide good support for the feet. Instruct your athletes to try on shoes in the afternoon, when the feet are swollen, to ensure accurate sizing. Remind them to wear the same number and type of socks that they would wear in practice and games.

Athletic shoes should be fitted to the length of the athlete's arch rather than to the length of the foot. The ball of the big toe should be directly over the widest part of the shoe when the athlete is standing. If the ball of the big toe falls in front of this point, the shoe is too short. An abnormal crease in the upper part of the shoe along the inner arch will tell you if this is the case. The break of the shoe—where it bends on push-off—should be at the widest part of the shoe.

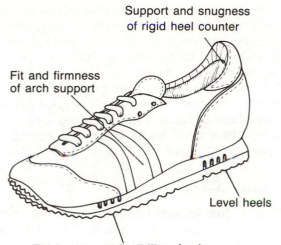

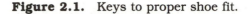

Figure 2.1. Keys to proper shoe fit.

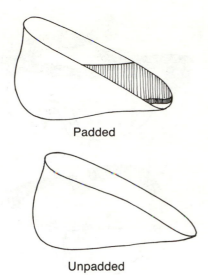

Commercially available heel cups

Figure 2.2. Padded and unpadded plastic heel cups.

Always have the athlete check the shoes on both feet since one foot may be larger than the other. Fit the shoes to the longer foot. The bottom line is this: If the shoe is not comfortable, it does not fit. You cannot break it in. Trying to do so causes blisters, corns, and calluses.

Care of Athletic Shoes. It is important that your athletes learn how to care for their shoes. The most common problem is with shoes that become saturated with water some time during the season. To allow for drying that will produce the least amount of deterioration, athletes should fill each shoe with crumpled paper and allow it to dry slowly, whether the shoe is made of leather, canvas, or nylon. They should apply a coating of saddle soap to leather shoes when drying is complete.

Tell your athletes that they should never wash athletic shoes in a washing machine or dry them in a dryer, both of which hasten the deterioration of the shoe materials, including the fabric and the bonding between layers.

Heel Protection. Some running shoes have a plastic heel cup built into the shoe as a counter-measure against repetitive pounding on the heel during running. While this is a good preventive measure, it is not adequate protection for a bruised heel. A vinyl foam heel pad cut to conform to the shape of the heel must be added to the heel cup to help dissipate and absorb force. Cut a hole in the pad to match the size and location of the tender area.

If the sport shoe you have selected does not have a heel cup, you can purchase one at many sporting goods stores. Select either a padded or unpadded cup (see Figure 2.2).

Because neither the heel cup nor the heel pad alone provides adequate protection for a bruised heel, we recommend a combination. For best results, supplement an unpadded heel cup with a ¼- to ⅜-inch-thick foam heel pad. If this method fails, it will be necessary to reduce the athlete's activity.

Corrective Lenses

Do not allow an athlete to wear prescription glasses for eye protection during activity unless the glasses are specifically designed for use in sports. Wire-rim frames and plain glass or plastic lenses are especially dangerous since they are not designed to withstand the stress of athletic activity. An accident could lead to a serious eye injury.

Prescription lenses should be ground of industrial plastic and set in either industrial or sports frames. An athlete may wear regular prescription glasses if a goggle with a Lexan-injected molded lens is worn over them.

Warn your athletes that contact lenses, both hard and soft, do not provide any protection for the eye, although the soft lenses will stay in place better. In activities in which eye protection is needed, the athlete who wears contact lenses also should wear some kind of protective eyewear.

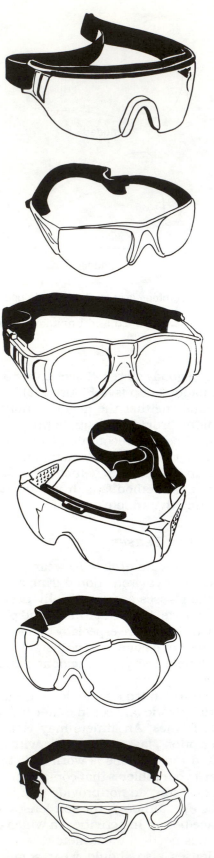

Figure 2.3. Varieties of protective eyewear.

In racquetball, squash, and handball, the wearing of eye guards should be compulsory. Athletes involved in racquet sports need to choose carefully among the different types of eye protectors that are available (see Figure 2.3). Look for an eye protector that does not limit peripheral vision yet offers good protection: Many of those without lenses will interfere with vision; some allow the eye to be struck by the ball.

Mouth Guards

Mouth guards are recommended for most contact/collision sports and play an important role in preventing cuts (lacerations) inside the mouth, fractured or loosened teeth, fractured or dislocated jaws, and concussions. Mouth guards work by distributing the force of a blow to all the teeth rather than localizing it at the point of contact. Coaches of contact/collision sports are wise to insist that their athletes wear mouth guards when participating in drills, scrimmages, or games.

You may find that some of your athletes dislike mouth guards (perhaps refusing to wear one) because they are uncomfortable or interfere with breathing and speech. In most cases, these problems are minimal and require you to explain that the discomfort is far outweighed by the protection they afford. You should check the athlete's mouth guard since the problem may be due to improper fitting. Remind the athlete that the mouth guard, like any piece of protective equipment, requires some "getting used to" before it will go unnoticed during play.

Types of Mouth Guards. There are two types of mouth guards generally used in sports:

- Mouth-formed (available commercially in junior and senior sizes)
- Custom-fit (molded by a dentist or oral surgeon)

Custom-fit mouth guards are more comfortable than are the commercial mouth-formed ones and tend to interfere less with breathing and speaking. When fitted properly, custom-fit mouth guards are tight enough to stay in place by themselves. However, they are more expensive. Custom-fit mouth guards are formed from a mold of the athlete's mouth. Consult a local dentist or oral surgeon about the cost.

The mouth-formed mouth guard, on the other hand, is briefly heated in boiling water, cooled to a working temperature, and then placed in the athlete's mouth so that the semipliable plastic can be molded to the athlete's bite. Such mouth guards are less expensive than custom-fit ones.

Athletes with braces; dental bridges, crowns (caps), or plates; missing or broken teeth; or odd-shaped dentition should use a custom-fit mouth guard.

If you have to trim a mouth guard for a better fit, do so very carefully (it is best to have the custom-fit one trimmed by a dental professional). Regardless of the type, mouth guards should be trimmed only to alleviate abnormal rubbing (the tips should be no shorter than the last molar). Too much trimming reduces the protective effectiveness of the mouth guard and may reduce its size to the point where it could be swallowed and become an airway obstruction.

Care of Mouth Guards. Like any other piece of equipment, a well-cared-for mouth guard will last the adult athlete several years. Children, because of the eruption of new teeth and general growth, may be limited to a particular mouth guard for one season (sometimes less). The child athlete who is erupting permanent teeth should follow the advice of his or her dentist or oral surgeon regarding mouth guards.

There are four major rules for the care of mouth guards:

- Store the mouth guard in a liquid solution. If the mouth guard manufacturer does not recommend any particular solution, ask a dentist for guidance. If the mouth guard is rinsed daily with a disinfectant mouthwash, it will be kept odor free and clean.
- Keep the mouth guard in its carrying case when traveling to and from practices and events.
- Avoid chewing on the mouth guard.
- Discard the mouth guard at the first sign of wear and have a new one molded.

It is a good idea to carry a few spare commercial mouth guards on trips so that you can mold a new one if needed. Do not give a commercial mouth guard to an athlete who has been told to wear a custom-fit one.

Physical Conditioning

When the athlete is poorly conditioned, the risk of injury is greatly increased. Unless the athlete has the necessary strength, endurance (both muscular and cardiorespiratory), and flexibility, the stresses placed on the body during participation may lead to injury. The coach must emphasize the importance of conditioning as it applies to playing the sport and preventing injuries. Some athletes will resist conditioning programs and will instead want to concentrate on skill development. These athletes require special attention to learn the value of proper conditioning.

Your conditioning programs should include specific exercises designed for preseason, season, and off-season conditioning. In the case of prepubertal children, endurance training does not significantly increase endurance capabilities. These children would benefit from training that is more oriented toward skills.

The adult "weekend athlete" is most often in need of exercises to improve flexibility and cardiorespiratory endurance. For guidelines on creating training programs, consult the *Coaches Guide to Sport Physiology* (Sharkey, 1986).

The Warm-Up

This is a set of exercises designed to be performed prior to activity. The typical program should be 5-15 minutes in length, with the exercises being done at a slow pace. The number of repetitions will depend on the physical condition of the athlete and the particular sport. The advantage of the warm-up is that it reduces muscle strain by improving circulation to deep muscles and improves flexibility through static stretching. Many athletes find that the warm-up helps to reduce the emotional stress that often precedes competition by providing a purposeful activity. Today the focus of this generalized warm-up is on stretching rather than calisthenics, as it has been in the past.

For most sports, a 15-minute warm-up routine should include the following:

- Easy running in place, jogging, or easy running for at least 5 minutes

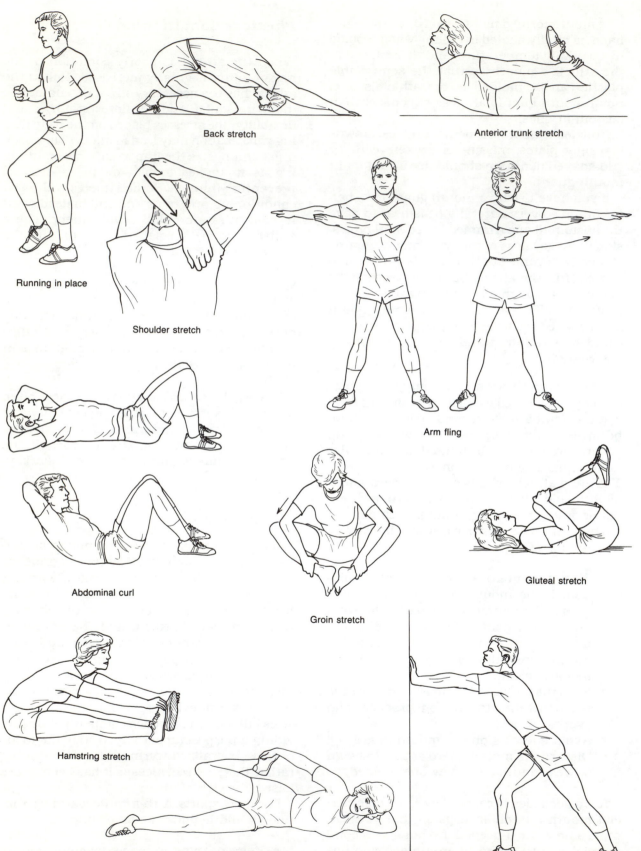

Running in place

Back stretch

Anterior trunk stretch

Shoulder stretch

Arm fling

Abdominal curl

Groin stretch

Gluteal stretch

Hamstring stretch

Quadriceps stretch

Calf stretch

Figure 2.4. Suggested stretching activities for inclusion in warm-up routines.

- A back-stretch exercise (useful in all sports due to the number of people with back problems)
- A trunk-stretch exercise (generally recommended for all sports)
- A shoulder-stretch exercise (usually not required of hurdlers, sprinters, and long-distance runners)
- An arm-fling exercise (usually not required of cyclists or long-distance runners; should be done slowly so that muscles are stretched, not torn)
- A modified sit-up—the abdominal curl (useful in all sports due to the number of back injuries that occur and the incidence of poor posture)
- A groin-stretch exercise (generally recommended for all sports)
- A gluteal-stretch exercise (generally recommended for all sports)
- A hamstring-stretch exercise (generally recommended for all sports)
- A quadricep-stretch exercise (generally recommended for all sports)
- A calf-stretch exercise (generally recommended for all sports)

Figure 2.4 shows an example of each of these exercises. General warm-up exercises should always be followed by simple warm-up activities that apply to the specific sport, for example, practice swings and throws for baseball and jogging followed by light strides and practice starts for track.

As you ask your athletes to warm up and stretch out, be sure to follow these guidelines:

- Begin with a general warm-up activity, such as walking or jogging.
- Stretches should be sustained. Do *not* bounce.
- Stretch the muscles until you feel a comfortable pulling sensation. You should *not* feel any quivering of the muscles.
- Hold the stretched position for 10 to 15 seconds.
- Relax as you stretch.

The Cool-Down

This program allows the athlete to bring body temperature, heart rate, and breathing to normal levels comfortably. Some experts believe that the cool-down period is more important than the warm-up in preventing injuries. The typical cool-down consists of jogging followed by walking until the heart rate is within 20 beats of the resting rate or the athlete has caught his or her breath. Stretching exercises should also be included in the cool-down regardless of the sport. In addition, many athletes find that the cool-down helps to reduce the emotional stress of competition, which helps reduce tension on neck and back muscles.

SUMMARY AND RECOMMENDATIONS

A sport-injury prevention program attempts to reduce the number of minor injuries and eliminate the more serious ones. The program should concentrate on medical support, the athlete's attitude, a safe environment, protective equipment, and physical conditioning.

1. The coach's approach to injury prevention should be a positive one. For example, the preseason physical can be used to guide athletes into activities that meet their physical needs, allow opportunities for success, and present little chance of injury. Perhaps the best approach for one athlete is the standard sport program. For another athlete, a special program of conditioning or a modified sport program may be needed to allow this athlete to reach his or her highest potential safely.

2. It is a coach's responsibility to develop in the athlete a positive attitude toward injury prevention that is present at all times, including when the athlete is on the sidelines or waiting to participate.

3. A safe environment means that all playing surfaces, pools, apparatus, and equipment are of an acceptable quality, clean, and in a good state of repair. A safe environment includes the proper protection for the specific sport and avoiding overexposure to excessive heat or cold, sun, and other potentially harsh environmental conditions.

4. The risk of injury is greatly increased if an athlete is poorly conditioned. Preseason, season, and off-season conditioning programs must be developed for each athlete. A warm-up and cool-down routine should be part of every conditioning program.

PART II
Emergency Care of Sport Injuries

Chapter 3

Assessing the Athlete for Injuries and Medical Emergencies

The coach may need to do the initial assessment of the athlete to determine the nature and extent of injury or sudden illness. The following sources of information must be considered:

- The preseason physical
- The athlete
- Bystanders
- The scene
- The cause of the injury
- Any information gained by examining the athlete

Prior to an athlete's participation in practice or an event, you should know if the athlete currently has or has ever had a particular medical problem. For example, the knowledge of a past joint injury may alert you to possible reinjury in situations where a blow to the joint does not usually produce any obvious injury requiring immediate care.

The best source of information as to what may be wrong is often the athlete. Asking the appropriate questions and listening closely to the answers usually will direct you to the specific problem. Keep in mind that the athlete may be unconscious, disoriented, or in too much pain to answer your questions. Others who have witnessed the injury as well as family members who are at the scene can provide information about how the injury occurred or what problems were noticed prior to the events that led to the injury. For example, the

athlete may have appeared to be dizzy prior to a fall.

If you did not witness the incident, the scene of an accident often will provide you with clues to the nature and possible cause of an injury. Look around and see if there are any objects that may have struck or been struck by the athlete. Is the playing surface smooth and uninterrupted? Are there any indications of something having recently been ingested to which the athlete was hypersensitive? Is the problem possibly related to the temperature at the scene?

Knowing what caused the injury (the *mechanism of injury*) can direct you to detect specific problems and additional injuries. The person who will be responsible to provide initial on-field injury assessment and care (coach, trainer, or assistant coach) should carefully observe the event while it is in progress, allowing the care provider to know how the injury occurred. If it is your responsibility to conduct assessments, then you must observe the athletes during practice and games.

During assessment, ask yourself these questions: What were the forces that caused the injury? Could damage have been caused directly by these forces? Are there usually injuries associated indirectly with the application of force (e.g., the athlete has fallen on his outstretched hand and has transferred the force to the bones of the elbow)? Were there any twisting forces involved (e.g., the force of the blow struck at the knee, but with the foot planted so that the leg twisted above the knee)? Is there more than one source of force being applied (e.g., the athlete was struck in the leg and then shoved to the ground, or his shoulder struck the ground first and then his head struck the ground or an object on the ground)? Basically, you must consider what caused the injury and what injuries typically occur under such circumstances. Common mechanisms of injury and their resulting injuries are outlined in Table 3.1.

The early emphasis in this book will be on the information you can gather by examining the athlete so that you can develop an understanding of injuries and gain the knowledge you need to ask the required questions and to look for specific clues that will help to assess the athlete. By the time you are ready to apply your knowledge in a coaching situation, you must be able to use each of the sources of assessment information as it applies to your specific situation in order to determine both the seriousness of the athlete's problem and the correct course of action to take.

THE ELEMENTS OF ASSESSMENT

During an assessment, you are trying to

- do no harm (the assessment procedures should not cause additional injury);
- detect life threatening emergencies;
- detect problems that may become life threatening;
- detect problems that need immediate care;

- detect problems requiring additional medical attention; and
- detect problems that require the athlete to be excluded from activity.

The assessment of an athlete for injury and illness consists of the primary survey and the secondary survey. The primary survey is concerned with the "ABCs" of emergency care:

A = **Airway** (the actions taken to ensure an open airway and adequate breathing)

B = **Breathing** (the actions taken to ensure adequate air exchange)

C = **Circulation** (the actions taken to ensure adequate circulation, the control of profuse bleeding, and the initial steps taken to control the development of shock)

The secondary survey is designed to detect problems that may become life threatening or may cause additional injury if allowed to go undetected and untreated.

THE PRIMARY SURVEY

In most cases, you will not have to perform a formal primary survey. The survey may be limited to detecting profuse bleeding, and usually, simple visual observation will tell you if the athlete is conscious and breathing. Most problems faced by the coach require only an interview and a limited physical examination. However, the primary survey is required when the athlete is unconscious, regardless of the possible cause of the unconsciousness. Whether or not you provide a full primary sur-

Table 3.1
Common Mechanisms of Injury

Mechanism	Injury
Direct blow	Contusions, sprains, dislocations, fractures
Binding force	Fractures, epiphyseal separations
Stretching force	Sprains, strains
Twisting force	Sprains, fractures
Muscular incoordination	Strains, sprains
Overuse	Tendinitis, bursitis, strains, sprains, shin splints, stress fractures, overuse syndromes

vey, remember that it is essential that an open airway be maintained.

During the primary survey, you are trying to determine quickly if there is a life-threatening problem and then provide the appropriate care to correct the problem. The coach should conduct a complete primary survey whenever the athlete is unconscious or has a low level of awareness. The steps for the primary survey are listed below; specific procedures are covered in the basic life-support skills presented in chapter 4.

You may need to do two things at once during the primary survey if profuse bleeding is evident. Have someone assist you with the care procedures. The first priority of emergency care is to establish an open airway. However, profuse bleeding cannot be allowed to go uncontrolled. You may have to establish an open airway and then stabilize the athlete's head in a tilted position while you control life-threatening bleeding. One person can usually establish and ensure the airway while another controls the bleeding.

WARNING:

Do *not* use the head-tilt method if the athlete is unconscious or has a possible spinal injury. In that instance, use the jaw-thrust method of opening the airway (see p. 38).

When conducting a primary survey, you should follow these procedures:

1. Determine if the athlete is responsive by *gently* tapping the athlete's shoulder and shouting, "Are you okay?" Although it is not part of most standards, it is a good idea to follow this statement with, "Don't move!" in case the athlete has a low level of awareness and tries to get up.
2. If the athlete can respond to your voice and tapping, he or she is breathing and is circulating blood (see Figure 3.1). If an athlete is not responsive, call out to someone who is at the scene and tell them to prepare to phone the EMS system.
3. Properly position the athlete when required. If the athlete does not respond to your voice and tapping *and* if you cannot detect adequate breathing, the athlete will have to be repositioned on

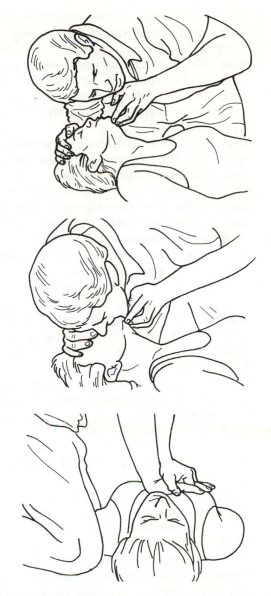

Figure 3.1. Check for respiration and circulation.

his or her back. This is done by a simple log-roll procedure that is described on page 166. Remember that moving the athlete's body is dangerous because of possible spinal injury. *Reposition the athlete only when you must do so to ensure a proper primary survey and to provide basic life-support procedures.*

4. Ensure an open airway and determine if breathing is adequate. If the athlete's problem is due to illness or injury not involving the spinal cord, the American Heart Association and the American Red Cross recommend using the head-tilt/chin-lift procedure as described on page

38. This maneuver is employed to provide the maximum airway opening.

5. If the athlete is unconscious, assume that there are spinal injuries present and use the jaw thrust as described on page 38. Regardless of the procedure used, the athlete must be lying flat on his or her back.

6. Once the airway is opened, ensure adequate breathing by using the look-listen-feel approach. Place your face close to the athlete's face and watch the chest. Look for the chest movements associated with air exchange, listen for the sounds of air being exchanged at the nose and mouth, and feel for air being exhaled through the nose and mouth.

7. If you detect an airway obstruction or if the athlete is not breathing, take immediate action. See chapter 4 for the detailed procedures for clearing the airway and providing rescue breathing (pulmonary resuscitation).

8. Check for indications of circulation. If the athlete is not breathing and you have opened the airway and have supplied artificial ventilations (two full breaths and the athlete is still not breathing), determine if there is a carotid pulse (see pp. 41-42).

9. If the athlete is unconscious, not breathing, and does not have a carotid pulse, begin cardiopulmonary resuscitation (CPR).

10. Once you are certain whether or not the unconscious athlete has a carotid pulse, have the person standing by call the EMS system. If the EMS dispatch knows that there is an unconscious patient who does not have a carotid pulse, an advanced life-support unit may be sent rather than a standard response team.

11. Detect profuse bleeding. Carefully look and feel for profuse bleeding. Avoid moving the athlete. Worry only about blood that is pulsating or flowing freely from wounds. This bleeding will have to be controlled as described in chapter 5.

12. If you are providing CPR and it causes profuse bleeding from open wounds, someone else will have to attempt to control this blood loss safely while you continue with CPR.

13. Begin to treat for shock. Unless resuscitation is being provided or the athlete's problem is due to exposure to excessive heat (e.g., heat stroke), cover his or her body to conserve body heat. This is the first step in controlling the development of shock. Other actions, such as elevating the athlete's legs, must be delayed until you have completed the secondary survey.

THE SECONDARY SURVEY

There are three parts to the secondary survey: the subjective interview, the gathering of vital signs, and the objective (physical) examination. The secondary survey concerns gathering information about the following:

- *Symptoms.* Symptoms might include pain, dizziness, chills, nausea, pressure, discomfort, the inability to use a limb fully, and a loss of feeling in a body part. Interview techniques are used to collect symptoms.
- *Signs.* Signs are the physical evidence that you collect while examining the athlete, for example, what you see, feel, hear, and smell. You may note bruises, swellings, areas that are tender to the touch, odd breath odors, an unusual sound made when the athlete moves a limb, or anything unusual gathered by using your senses.
- *Vital signs.* At the level of care that is provided by the coach, vital signs include the athlete's level of awareness, pulse rate and character (rhythm and force), breathing rate and character (rhythm and depth), and relative skin temperature and color. The specifics on each of these vital signs will be covered later in this chapter.

The Interview

Keep in mind that most people truly believe that "actions speak more loudly than words." During the typical interview it is possible to begin to assess certain problems visually. When you do so, make certain that you keep contact with what the athlete is saying. Do not turn away either while asking questions or while listening to responses. The interview is usually limited to a few key questions. The interview, however, may become more complex when the injury is severe, when you must depend on bystanders' answers, when you do not personally know the athlete, or when you did not witness the events leading to the injury.

Try to ask some questions that are open ended, or that allow the other person to provide the details he or she believes are important. Your other questions should be worded so that the response gives you a specific piece of information. As you learn more about the nature of illnesses and injuries, specific questions to ask will become more evident.

When you have completed the interview, you should know the following:

- The athlete's name
- The athlete's age
- The chief complaint (what is wrong)
- How the problem occurred (what happened)
- If there are other complaints
- If there were preexisting problems
- If the athlete has been seeing a physician
- If any medications are being taken and what they are
- If there are any allergies (included in the athlete's preseason examination record)

Because of your relationship with team members, you may already have much of this information. Be sure to ask for information you are unable to gather from previous contact.

Vital Signs

The vital signs of level of awareness, pulse, respiration, and relative skin temperature and color should be gathered more than once during the assessment. This evaluation is the only way to detect improvement, decline, or a steady state in the athlete's condition. For example, following an injury, an adult athlete (over the age of 18) has a breathing rate of 30 breaths per minute. After you have completed other elements of the assessment, a second gathering of vital signs may indicate a breathing rate of 15 breaths per minute (in the normal range of 12-20). This is an improvement and is usually significant. However, if the breathing rate stayed at 30 per minute or increased, then you are dealing with an emergency that requires the help of a physician as soon as possible.

Taking a second set of vital signs can be very important for certain types of injury, including possible fractures and internal bleeding. The bodies of many athletes under the age of 35 can delay the development of shock by changing heart rate and blood-vessel diameter (compensated shock). The delay can last for 5 or more minutes until the compensation is lost or no longer adequate. At that point, severe shock develops quickly.

The first evaluation of vital signs may indicate a minor or moderate problem when, in fact, the nature of the problem is very serious. Additional observations and the gathering of vital signs will alert you to the true severity of the athlete's problem.

If the nature of the athlete's problem is a sudden illness or a difficulty related to a known condition, vital signs should be gathered during the interview *and* after the physical examination. Depending on the nature of the problem, additional or continuous assessments of vital signs may be required.

A serious injury or any case involving an unconscious athlete also requires that vital signs be taken both before and after the physical examination. When the athlete's problem is a minor injury, the assessment of vital signs can be delayed until after the physical examination.

Level of Awareness

Your assessment of the athlete's level of awareness begins with the primary survey and continues through assessment and care. You should keep track of this by the "AVPU" method, which requires you to consider the following:

A = **Alertness and orientation** (Does the athlete know what is happening?)

V = **Verbal awareness** (Can the athlete respond to your voice?)

P = **Painful stimuli** (Does the athlete who does not respond to your voice withdraw from a painful stimulus such as being pinched on the back of the hand?)

U = **Unconsciousness** (Is the athlete totally unresponsive?)

Always report any changes in the athlete's level of awareness. If the athlete was unconscious and then regains consciousness, make certain that the EMS system is informed. It is very important that the EMTs know whether the athlete regains consciousness and then suffers another loss of consciousness.

Pulse

The pulse that is used in determining vital signs is the wrist, or *radial pulse*. Figure 3.2 illustrates the positioning of the fingertips for the radial pulse. When no pulse can be detected at the wrists, a *carotid pulse* rate should be measured (see pp. 41-42).

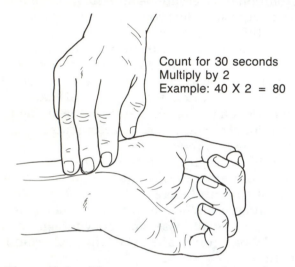

Count for 30 seconds
Multiply by 2
Example: 40 X 2 = 80

Figure 3.2. The proper way to evaluate the radial pulse.

To locate and assess the radial pulse, take the following steps:

1. Working on the palm side of the hand, place the tips of your first three fingers on the crease between the hand and the wrist that is found on the thumb side of the wrist. Do *not* use your own thumb as it has a pulse of its own, and you would be measuring your own pulse rate.
2. Apply pressure with these three fingertips to feel the pulse beats. You may have to increase the pressure applied if the pulse is weak. If you keep all three fingers in contact with the athlete's wrist, you will not need to apply much pressure.
3. Count the number of beats for 30 seconds and multiply this number by 2 to determine the number of beats per minute (pulse rate). If you are counting

the pulse beats and believe that the rate is probably very high or low, you should count the beats for 1 full minute to determine the rate.
4. As you count the beats, judge the character (strength) of the pulse.
5. Have someone record your results and note the time the assessment was done.

Pulse character consists of the rhythm and force of the pulse. As you count the beats, note whether the pulse rhythm is regular or irregular and whether the pulse feels strong (full) or weak (thready).

What is considered to be the "normal," or at-rest, pulse rate for an individual cannot be determined by looking at an average pulse rate for the entire population. The normal rate should be determined by assessing at-rest pulse during the preseason physical. The coach should make note of this rate for each athlete and try to confirm the preseason data by periodically reevaluating the pulse of each of your athletes while they are at rest. Any athlete who shows a marked change in pulse rate should be reassessed by a physician.

General guidelines for the pulse rate of adults should be followed in emergencies:

- A rate above 100 beats per minute is rapid and above 120 beats per minute is very serious.
- Once the rate exceeds 150 beats per minute, consider the athlete to have a life threatening condition.
- Any pulse rate below 60 beats per minute must be considered to be slow unless the individual is a well-conditioned athlete (some have rates as low as 40 beats per minute).
- Regardless of the condition of the person, the pulse rate should not be more than a few beats per minute below the rate of the preparticipation physical.

Guidelines for adolescents include the following:

- Most adolescents (12-18 years of age) should have a pulse rate in the range of 70-85 beats per minute. Their recovery rate is usually very rapid.
- Any rate that stays 10 beats per minute above or below the at-rest figure must be considered to be a sign of injury or illness.

For children between the ages of 5 and 12, the pulse rate should fall into the range of 60-120 beats per minute, with the rate slowing as the child grows older.

Exertion, reactions to pain, and apprehension will markedly affect the pulse rate, and you should keep these factors in mind during your first assessment. As the athlete rests, the pulse rate should quickly return to the athlete's typical range. If it does not, assume that there is something wrong that will require additional assessment by someone with more training.

Breathing Rate and Character

Many people will change their breathing rate if they know that someone is monitoring it. So, when you have finished measuring the athlete's pulse rate, keep your fingers on his or her wrist until you have completed your determination of the breathing rate, then record the pulse rate after you have finished assessing breathing. By taking this approach, the athlete will probably be unaware that you are assessing his or her breathing.

The breathing rate is determined by watching the chest movements associated with adequate breathing. One breath is one inhalation (inspiration) and one exhalation (expiration) combined. Many males show a pronounced chest movement at the level of the diaphragm, while many females show it at the level of the collarbones. To determine the breathing rate, count the number of breaths for 30 seconds and multiply by 2. If you believe that the rate will be very high or low, count for 1 full minute to determine the number of breaths per minute.

There will be times when you cannot determine the breathing rate by watching chest movements (e.g., during shallow breathing). When this happens, tell the athlete that you must touch the lower end of the breastbone. Keep your hand resting lightly in this position and count the number of breaths to determine the breathing rate.

While you are determining the breathing rate, note if the athlete's breathing rhythm is regular or irregular, if the breathing is done with ease or difficulty, if breathing is shallow or deep, and if any unusual noises can be heard that are associated with breathing.

The at-rest breathing rate for the athlete should be determined during the preseason physical and periodically reevaluated by the coach. The general guidelines for breathing rates for adults are as follows:

- The breathing rate is 12-20 breaths per minute, with most individuals having a rate of 12-15 breaths per minute.
- Once the rate reaches and stays at 28 or more breaths per minute, the person must be considered to have a serious emergency.

For adolescents:

- The range is 16-20 breaths per minute, with 16-18 per minute being the range for those 15-18 years of age.
- The same emergency figures used for adults are usually applied to adolescent breathing rates.

For children:

- By the time a child is between the ages of 5 and 10, the high rates found in infancy and early childhood fall to 24 breaths per minute.
- A rate at or above 36 breaths per minute is a true emergency for any child 5-12 years of age.

As with the pulse rate, the breathing rate is influenced by exertion, the initial reaction to pain, and apprehension. More than one assessment will be necessary. If the rate does not quickly fall into the normal range as the athlete rests, then you must assume that there is a serious problem requiring assessment by a more highly trained individual.

Relative Skin Temperature and Color

The temperature and condition of the skin can give valuable clues about the nature and severity of an injury or illness. The detection of hot, dry skin may point the way to detecting heat stroke. Cool and clammy skin may indicate the development of shock. Always determine the athlete's relative skin temperature by placing the back of your hand lightly against his or her forehead (if there are no injuries in this region and there are no possible spinal injuries). Determine if the skin temperature feels normal, warm, hot, cool, or cold. Also note whether the skin feels dry, wet, or clammy.

Throughout the physical examination, be aware of any changes in skin temperature and condition. Note whether one part of the body feels significantly colder or warmer than other areas (e.g., the abdominal wall feels hot). Pay particular attention to the skin temperature on an injured limb. Does the skin feel cooler past the injury site (closer to an extremity)? This could mean that the blood flow has been interrupted. Does one limb feel cooler or warmer than the same limb on the opposite side of the body? This could indicate circulatory or nerve damage. Is the skin a different color (red, pale, ashen, or blue) than normal?

The Physical Examination

This examination as it applies to prehospital emergency care may be limited or complete, depending on the nature of the injury, potential injuries associated with detected injuries, and the training of the individual who is doing the examination. A complete examination, to the level of your training, is required for an unconscious injured athlete if specific care is to be rendered. Remember that any unconscious, injured athlete must be assumed to have spinal injuries. Usually, a coach can be expected only to do a primary survey, control bleeding, begin treating for shock, and protect the athlete while waiting for more highly trained personnel to arrive. If you are without a trainer and your athletes will be participating in areas where an EMS response or other quick, on-the-scene care cannot be provided, you must receive additional training above the basic first aid level (e.g., advanced first aid and emergency care or First Responder certification).

A limited examination would be appropriate for situations in which the athlete is alert, the injury is probably not very serious, the force causing the injury was not great, and you witnessed the event. The examination can usually be limited if the nature of the problem is known to be a preexisting medical problem, such as asthma, and there are no injuries.

Preparing for a Physical Examination

Regardless of the extent of the examination, always ask the alert athlete if you can touch a given area of the body. Warn the athlete of the possibility of pain being produced during each phase of the examination.

Remove only the articles of clothing that must be removed to expose an injury site and lift or cut away clothing that blocks your view

of a suspected injury. Do not pull off clothing as this may cause additional injury.

Unless you are trained to do so, do not attempt to remove a helmet from the head of an athlete who may have head, facial, neck, shoulder, or spinal injuries. More will be said about the dangers of helmet removal in chapter 12.

Do not attempt to remove form-fitting gloves as this may cause additional injury and may restart bleeding that wearing the glove was controlling.

Unless you suspect that an injury needs immediate care, do not remove shoes, as this may cause additional harm to fractures of the pelvis, ankle, foot, or lower limb and may restart controlled bleeding.

The Limited Examination

Do not be too quick to limit the physical examination and be sure you are dealing with a problem that allows for a limited examination. Television instant replays have shown that some injuries occur differently than most people believe. These same replays have shown that many secondary problems (e.g., head and neck injuries) are possible during most falls and contact-sport injuries.

In most cases, you will be able to use a limited interview and examination to determine the nature of the athlete's problem. You should make it a habit to scan the athlete's entire body quickly in case there may be a second problem. Also, remember to assess areas adjacent to the affected area. For example, if the arm is mildly injured, there still may be problems with the shoulder and elbow. Depending on the nature of the problem, your limited examination should consider the following:

- *Obvious injury or deformity.* This includes bruises, swelling or hardness (under the skin or in the abdomen), cuts, and deformity of size, shape, or length.
- *Tenderness or pain.* This includes point tenderness and pain only on movement as reported by the athlete. (Do not have the athlete move an injured body part to confirm that the pain is still present. Complete your assessment and have the athlete keep the injured part immobilized.) Point tenderness is a painful reaction to mild pressure applied to the site by the fingertips.

- *Discoloration.* This is indicated by reddening, bruise coloration (ecchymosis), blanching (turning white), or blue discoloration or cyanosis (associated with failing circulation).
- *Loss of use.* This is indicated by the limited or complete loss of function or range of motion.
- *Guarding.* The athlete will attempt to hold the injured part or not use the part.
- *Noises.* This includes any grating, popping, snapping, or cracking sounds under the skin during movement or at the time of injury as well as unusual breathing noises (e.g., wheezing).
- *Unusual or false motion.* The athlete will show restricted or improper body mechanics, exaggerated or unproper motion at a joint, or false motion at an injury site on the shaft of the bone (e.g., there is movement in the upper arm as if the arm bone, or humerus, had a joint between the elbow and the shoulder).
- *Loss of distal pulse.* The pulse at the far, or distal, end of a limb cannot be felt.
- *Loss of nerve function.* The athlete cannot tell you which digit is touched, cannot wave a hand or wiggle a foot, or cannot push against your hand with his or her foot or grasp your hand with his or her hand. The athlete may report numbness or a tingling sensation.
- *Skin temperature changes.* An area of the body may feel hot or cool, one limb may be warmer or cooler than the same limb on the other side of the body, or a limb may be cooler closer to an extremity than the injury site.

During a limited examination, it is essential that you examine the injured areas as well as those that adjoin the site of injury. If a conscious athlete has an injury to the upper arm, then you must examine the entire extremity, including the shoulder. The adjoining areas of the chest and back must also be examined for possible injury.

SUMMARY AND RECOMMENDATIONS

The coach who is responsible for the initial care of injured and sick athletes must know how to conduct a proper assessment. Information can be gained from the athlete, bystanders, the scene, mechanism of injury, and a physical examination of the athlete.

1. The assessment consists of a primary survey, the gathering of vital signs, and a secondary survey.
2. The primary survey is concerned with assessing the athlete's state of awareness, airway, breathing, and circulation.
3. The vital signs to consider are state of awareness, pulse rate and character, breathing rate and character, and relative skin temperature and color.
4. The secondary survey consists of the subjective interview and the objective (physical) examination.
5. You must be prepared to conduct a limited physical examination. The factors to consider in the limited examination are shown in Figure 3.3. Remember, you must consider any injured, unconscious athlete to have spinal injuries, and the athlete will need a complete assessment by someone more highly trained.

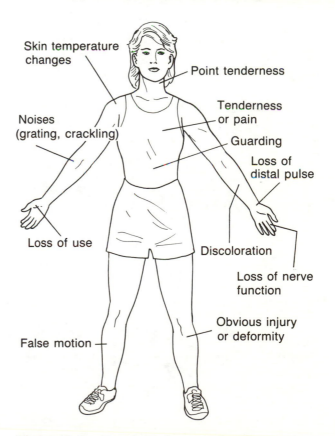

Figure 3.3. Factors to be considered in a limited examination.

Chapter 4
Basic Life Support

Airway obstruction, the cessation of breathing (respiratory arrest), and the stopping of heart action (cardiac arrest) are not common in sports, especially when the athletes are children, adolescents, or young adults. However, they do occur, and are often linked to undetected respiratory and heart problems, foreign objects in the airway (e.g., mouth guards or gum), or the coach's sensitivity to the effects of the environmental conditions. As a coach, you must be prepared for these emergencies and be able to initiate life-saving procedures as quickly as possible.

The information presented in this chapter is based on the basic cardiac life-support courses offered by the American Heart Association and the American Red Cross and is *not* a substitute for taking these courses. You should have certification in basic cardiac life support from one of these organizations. Because these skills require practice and because changes are periodically made in the procedures applied, it is recommended that you be recertified every year.

THE ABCs OF EMERGENCY CARE

As explained in chapter 3, the primary survey considers the problems that are critical to the life of the athlete. Traditionally, these problems and the steps taken to provide care are known as the ABCs of emergency care:

A = **Airway**

B = **Breathing**

C = **Circulation**

Basic cardiac life support considers each of these functions and allows the rescuer to open and maintain the airway, to ensure adequate breathing or provide rescue breathing (pulmonary resuscitation) and to ensure adequate circulation or provide cardiopulmonary resuscitation (CPR).

These measures can be successful because there is a difference between clinical and biological death. *Clinical death* occurs when the person stops breathing and his or her heart stops circulating blood; it may be reversed if oxygen can be circulated to the brain and advanced life-support measures provided. *Biological death* occurs when the brain cells die and is irreversible. Approximately 4-6 minutes after someone stops breathing and circulating blood, lethal changes may take place in the brain. Approximately 10 minutes after clinical death, brain cells start to die. The times vary slightly because of age (it takes longer for lethal changes and brain-cell death in infants and young children) or because the environment has drastically lowered body temperature (e.g., cold-water drowning). However, the sooner basic cardiac life-support steps are begun, the better the person's chances for survival.

Most people who are not in a hospital and who have been clinically dead for 10 minutes or more before basic cardiac life support is started cannot be resuscitated successfully. This is not to say that you should not begin basic cardiac life-support measures if the person has not been breathing for more than 10 minutes, but quick assessment and action are needed. In many cases, witnesses who report this information are inaccurate about when actual cardiac arrest took place. There have been instances in which people were successfully resuscitated even after 10 minutes of confirmed clinical death.

HEART-LUNG-BRAIN FUNCTION

There is a close relationship between the functions of the heart, lungs, and brain. Basically, if one fails, soon all three will fail. If someone's heart stops beating, he or she will stop breathing, usually within 30 seconds. Biological death will soon follow as the brain cells are deprived of oxygen. If a person stops breathing, the lack of oxygen will affect the heart and the brain. Cardiac arrest will develop, and biological death will usually occur within 10 minutes. In some instances, a head injury may be severe enough to cause damage to the respiratory and/or cardiac control centers of the brain. Inefficient heart or respiratory function will follow, eventually leading to respiratory or cardiac failure, then arrest, and then biological death. This relationship, with one problem often leading to another, indicates that the sooner respiratory arrest or respiratory arrest and cardiac arrest are detected, and the sooner basic life support is started, the better the person's chances for survival.

The Respiratory System

Breathing is an involuntary act that is controlled by the respiratory centers in the brain. Signals are sent from the brain to contract the diaphragm and the muscles between the ribs to produce an inspiration. When these muscles relax, an expiration takes place.

The major structures of the respiratory system include the following (see Figure 4.1):

- *Nose*. This is the main passageway for air to enter and leave the respiratory system.
- *Mouth*. This is normally the secondary passageway for air to enter and leave the respiratory system. As the demand to rid the body of carbon dioxide increases, or when there is a greater need for oxygen, the mouth becomes the primary passageway for air exchange.
- *Pharynx*. This is most commonly called the throat and is the upper passageway shared by the respiratory and digestive

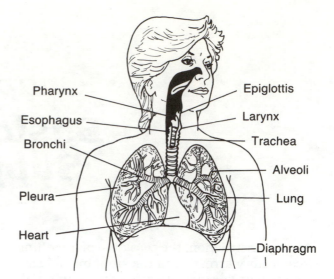

Figure 4.1. The respiratory system.

systems. Pieces of food may block this structure, thus obstructing the airway.
- *Larynx*. This is commonly referred to as the voice box and is the airway found in the neck that connects the throat and the trachea.
- *Trachea*. This structure, the windpipe, receives air from the voice box and carries it to the bronchial tree.
- *Bronchial tree*. These tubes branch out from the trachea and become smaller in size until the exchange levels of the lungs are reached.
- *Lungs*. These elastic organs contain most of the bronchial tree and the microscopic air sacs (alveoli), where oxygen is picked up from the lungs and carbon dioxide taken from the blood.

The Heart

The heart is a muscular pump that is situated in the center of the chest cavity and behind the breastbone (sternum). It is about the size of a person's fist, with the bulk of its mass positioned to the left of the body's midline. The right side of the heart receives blood from the body and sends it to the lungs to be oxygenated. The left side receives the oxygenated blood from the lungs and pumps the blood out to the entire body.

The typical adult, when at rest, will have 70 heart beats per minute, pumping 10 pints of blood during this time period. An adult male weighing 150 pounds has approximately 12 pints of blood. So, when at rest, over 85% of his blood is circulated completely every minute. During exercise, the typical adult heart can circulate up to 70 pints per minute. During the course of a lifetime, the heart will beat over 2.5 billion times, circulating 450 million pints of blood.

RESCUE BREATHING

Rescue breathing is the act of providing breaths of air to the lungs of a person who is experiencing respiratory arrest. This process is also called pulmonary resuscitation, or, more colloquially, artificial respiration. There are slight variations in technique between procedures for children and adults. According to American Heart Association guidelines, anyone from the ages of 1 to 8 should be treated as a child, and an individual over 8 years of age should be treated as an adult.

Many people ask how air that is being exhaled by a rescuer can be of any benefit to someone who is experiencing respiratory arrest. The air in the atmosphere is about 21% oxygen, while that being exhaled contains almost 16% oxygen, a reduction of 5%. This means that exhaled air still has more than three times the amount of oxygen that is normally removed by the lungs during a typical breath.

Detecting Respiratory Arrest

Before providing pulmonary resuscitation, you must take the following steps (see Figure 4.2):

1. *Establish unresponsiveness.* A person who is responsive does not need resuscitation. Gently shake the person's shoulder and loudly ask, "Are you OK?"
2. *Call out for help.* Make certain that someone else knows there is a problem. If you are alone, call out even if you do not believe anyone else is around—you may be mistaken. You will need another person to be prepared to phone for help, but delay this call until you can determine if you are dealing with respiratory or with cardiac arrest. Do not delay detecting breathlessness in order to find assistance.

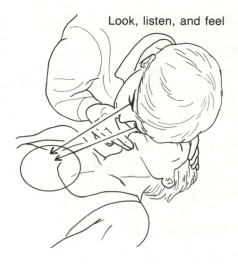

Look, listen, and feel

Figure 4.2. Detecting respiratory arrest.

3. *Reposition the person.* This repositioning is to be done *only* when you must move the athlete to determine if he or she is breathing or to provide basic life support. Begin by straightening the athlete's legs and positioning the athlete's arm that is closest to you above his or her head. Next, carefully cradle the athlete's head and neck with one of your hands and reach across the athlete to grasp the distant armpit. Steady the neck and pull at the armpit to roll the athlete, as a unit, onto his or her side. Finally, roll the athlete onto the back and reposition the extended arm.
4. *Open the airway.* Make certain that this is done in every case. Select the appropriate technique on the basis of presence or absence of head, neck, or back injuries. Two techniques are described on page 38.
5. *Establish breathlessness.* Use the look-listen-feel method. Position your ear over the person's nose and mouth as you look at the chest. Then,
   - *look* for the rise and fall of the chest that is associated with breathing,
   - *listen* for air being expired, and
   - *feel* for air being expired onto your cheek.
6. *Decide if the person is breathing.* Take at least 3, but no more than 5, seconds to determine whether the person is breathing. If the person is not breathing, you will have to initiate rescue breathing immediately.

Opening the Airway

The airway must be opened before proper assessment and rescue breathing can begin. The airway of an unconscious athlete often becomes obstructed by the tongue. If the coach applies a simple maneuver to move the lower jaw forward, the tongue, which is attached to the lower jaw, will be lifted away from the back of the throat. Two methods are commonly used to open the airway, the head tilt/chin lift and the jaw thrust.

Head Tilt/Chin Lift

This method is recommended for uninjured, unresponsive athletes who may be experiencing respiratory arrest or who are having problems breathing because of a possible airway obstruction. To apply this technique, you should do the following (see Figure 4.3):

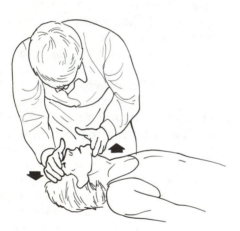

Figure 4.3. Opening the airway by using the head-tilt/chin-lift technique.

1. Make certain that the athlete is flat on his or her back.
2. Position yourself at the athlete's side at head level.
3. Use your hand closest to the athlete's chest to support the lower jaw and lift the chin. This is done by placing the fingers of your hand under the lower jaw at the bony prominence of the chin and using them to lift the chin forward. Do *not* allow your fingers to compress the soft tissues that are found under the chin as you could obstruct the airway. Do *not* use your thumb to lift the chin. Instead, the thumb can be used to de-

press the athlete's lower lip to improve the opening at the mouth.
4. Use your other hand to press gently on the athlete's forehead. This will help to tilt the head back.

If the athlete is a small child, you must be careful when applying the head tilt. Too great a tilt may partially close the airway. The tilt will be less than for an adult; however, you must ensure that the tilt is sufficient to supply an adequate airway.

The Jaw Thrust

This method is recommended for use on injured athletes and is the only technique approved for use on anyone suspected of having neck or spinal injuries. To apply this maneuver, take the following steps (see Figure 4.4):

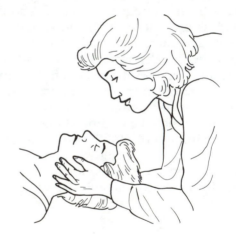

Figure 4.4. The jaw-thrust technique can be used for injured athletes. Do not tilt or rotate the head.

1. Properly position the athlete on the back, taking great care to protect the spine.
2. Position yourself at the athlete's head. Place your hands on each side of the athlete's lower jaw and rest your elbows on the same surface on which the athlete is lying. Next, grasp the angles of the athlete's lower jaw.
3. Use both hands to move the athlete's lower jaw forward. Apply most of the pressure with your index fingers, using your forearms to stabilize the head during the maneuver. Do *not* allow the head to rotate.

Providing Breaths

Note: The American Heart Association has recommended that emergency care personnel avoid direct contact with their patients' body fluids during rescue breathing. EMTs are trained to use pocket face masks and bag-valve-mask units that help prevent such contact. The use of these devices is not part of a coach's training or citizen-level training by the American Heart Association and American Red Cross. New devices that create a barrier between rescuer and patient yet allow for air exchange are being tested (e.g., Laerdal's Patient Face Shields). Contact your local American Heart Association or American Red Cross office and find out if these devices are now accepted for use by citizens and if training in their use is available.

The breaths delivered during rescue breathing should be provided so that the ventilation will cause the athlete's chest to rise. Too small a breath will not adequately ventilate the athlete, and too large a breath will force air into the stomach (see p. 44).

The Mouth-to-Mouth Technique

The most common method of providing ventilation is the mouth-to-mouth technique. To perform mouth-to-mouth ventilations when applying the head tilt/chin lift, follow this procedure:

1. Maintain an open airway, and, if necessary, clear the airway (pp. 47-48). For some sports, the athlete will be wearing a mouth guard. Any material in the mouth, including a loose mouth guard or one that obstructs the airway, must be removed.
2. Pinch the athlete's nostrils closed using the thumb and index finger of the hand that is on the forehead. It is best to pinch at the openings of the nostrils.
3. Make certain that there are no objects in your mouth (e.g., gum). Open your mouth wide and take a deep breath.
4. Keep your mouth open wide and place it around the athlete's mouth, forming a *tight* seal with your lips against the face. This does not require more than a light contact with the athlete. Many people at first apply too much pressure.

If the athlete is a small child, you may find it easier to cover both the nose and mouth with your mouth, eliminating the need to pinch the nostrils shut.

5. Exhale into the athlete's airway, looking to see that the chest rises and falls and feeling for resistance to the flow of your breath. You should take 1-1.5 seconds to deliver this breath smoothly. If your attempt to provide a breath fails, reposition the athlete's head and re-attempt the breath (see Figure 4.5).
6. After delivering the ventilation, break contact with the nose and mouth, turn your head toward the athlete's chest, and quickly take another breath. During this time, some air will passively flow from the victim's lungs. Listen for the passive exhalation.
7. Deliver this second breath in 1-1.5 seconds.
8. If the athlete does not begin to breathe on his or her own (spontaneous breathing), determine if he or she has a carotid pulse (see pp. 41-42). If no pulse is felt, you will have to initiate cardiopulmonary resuscitation (CPR). If the person has a pulse and is not breathing, you will have to continue with rescue breathing.
9. Alert the EMS system. Make certain that someone is assigned to tell the dispatcher whether the athlete has a pulse and whether he or she is breathing. In many areas of the country, having this information will allow the dispatcher to order an advanced cardiac life support unit rather than a typical EMS response.
10. If there is a pulse, continue with rescue breathing by

   - maintaining an open airway;
   - pinching the nostrils closed;
   - taking a deep breath;
   - forming the proper seal;
   - providing the ventilation as you watch the chest rise, taking 1-1.5 seconds per ventilation;
   - breaking contact to allow for a passive exhalation as you turn your head to watch the chest fall and listen and feel for the return of air; and
   - taking a deep breath to begin a new

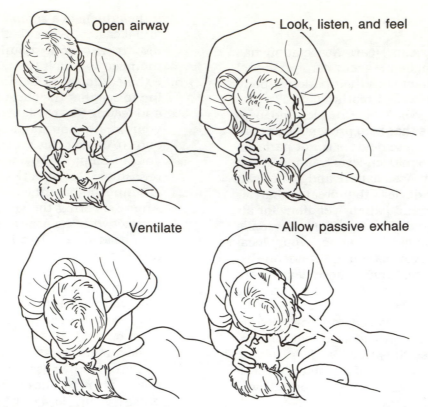

Open airway

Look, listen, and feel

Ventilate

Allow passive exhale

Figure 4.5.   Rescue breathing—the mouth-to-mouth technique.

cycle. For adult athletes, you should deliver *one breath every 5 seconds* so that the rate of ventilation is 12 breaths per minute. A child should receive *one breath every 4 seconds* so that the rate of ventilation is 15 breaths per minute.

11. Every couple of minutes, check for a carotid pulse (pp. 41-42). If there is a pulse, continue with rescue breathing. The absence of a pulse indicates that you will have to begin CPR.

Failure to apply the steps of the mouth-to-mouth technique properly will lead to poor ventilation by the victim. The most common mistakes made include the following:

- Failure to achieve a tight seal over the victim's mouth
- Failure to pinch the victim's nostrils closed
- Failure to open the airway properly
- Failure to have the victim's mouth opened wide enough to receive the ventilations

If you wear dentures, you may occasionally experience an additional problem. As you ventilate the athlete, the dentures may become loose and interfere with the delivery of breaths. This problem can usually be avoided by making light contact with the athlete's face when forming the seal as too much pressure may loosen the dentures. If light contact is being applied and there is still a problem with dentures loosening, use your tongue to help hold your upper denture in place.

If you are providing mouth-to-mouth ventilations to an injured athlete while using the jaw-thrust technique, you will not be able to release one hand from the jaw in order to close the nostrils. Rather, you will have to press your cheek against the nostrils to seal them shut during the delivery of each breath, which requires practice if it is to be effective during emergency conditions. Since a coach must be prepared to provide rescue breathing for the athlete who may have a spinal injury, you must learn to be efficient with mouth-to-mouth ventilations while applying the jaw thrust to open the airway.

The Mouth-to-Nose Technique

There are situations in which it is more appropriate to ventilate the athlete through the nose. The mouth-to-nose technique is preferred when there is severe mouth injury, when a lower-jaw injury prevents opening the mouth, when a proper seal around the mouth cannot be formed, and when an airway obstruction in the mouth cannot be cleared.

The procedures for this technique are very similar to those for the mouth-to-mouth technique. One hand is used to maintain a head tilt while the other hand is used to lift the lower jaw. In this case, the lift is done so that the mouth remains closed. To provide ventilations, you will need to take a deep breath and deliver the ventilation by sealing your mouth around the athlete's nose. Remember to feel for resistance and watch the chest rise. Then break contact with the victim's nose and allow for a passive exhalation. This process can be improved if you slightly open the athlete's mouth as he or she exhales. You must remember to close his or her mouth when you provide the next ventilation.

Ventilation rates are the same as for mouth-to-mouth ventilations: one breath every 5 seconds (12 per minute) for adults and one breath every 4 seconds (15 per minute) for children.

The jaw thrust can be used with the mouth-to-nose technique when there is the possibility of spinal injury. Care must be taken so that the lower lip does not retract as you push with your thumbs. If it does, sealing the athlete's mouth with your cheek will be much more difficult. Remember to release this seal to allow for passive exhalation.

CARDIOPULMONARY RESUSCITATION (CPR)

Cardiopulmonary resuscitation is used to prevent biological death when someone is experiencing cardiac arrest. The person will not be responsive, will not be breathing, and will not be circulating blood. The techniques applied during CPR provide the athlete with air and circulation.

The breaths delivered during CPR follow the same principle as those used during rescue breathing. They are delivered between a set number of external chest compressions that cause changes in pressure in the chest cavity that, in turn, force the blood to circulate. One-way valves in the heart and veins keep the blood circulating in its normal pattern.

Basic Techniques of CPR

The techniques used in CPR combine what you have learned about rescue breathing with the procedure for delivering external chest compressions. As with rescue breathing, slight modifications must be made when performing CPR on a child (1-8 years of age). Two-rescuer CPR, utilizing two persons to carry out CPR, is no longer recommended for the general public. As a result, only one-rescuer CPR will be considered in this book.

Starting CPR

The same procedures that are used for establishing the need for rescue breathing are followed when determining the need for CPR. You should follow these procedures (see Figure 4.6):

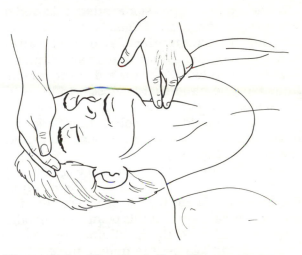

Figure 4.6. The signs of cardiac arrest: unresponsive, no breathing, no pulse.

1. Establish unresponsiveness.
2. Call out for help if you are working alone.
3. Properly position the athlete on a hard surface or the ground.
4. Establish an open airway.
5. Establish breathlessness by the look-listen-feel method.
6. Deliver two breaths, taking 1-1.5 seconds per breath.
7. Check for spontaneous breathing.
8. Take 5-10 seconds to check for a carotid pulse if the athlete is not breathing. To evaluate the carotid pulse, start by locating the athlete's Adam's apple (thyroid

cartilage). Place the tips of your index and middle fingers over the midline of this structure and slide them toward the side of the athlete's neck that is closest to you. Do not reach across the neck as this may lead to the improper application of finger pressure, which may close the athlete's airway. With the palm side of your fingertips on the side of the athlete's neck, apply gentle pressure to the area between the windpipe and the large muscle that makes up the side of the neck. You will not need to apply much pressure to feel the pulse. You should feel for 5-10 seconds to determine whether there is a pulse.

9. Have someone alert the EMS dispatcher.
10. Begin CPR if the athlete has no pulse.

The CPR Compression Site

External chest compressions *must* be delivered to a specific site on the athlete's chest. To find this site, kneel at the athlete's side with both of your knees on the ground or floor and pointing toward the athlete. Place the index and middle fingers of the hand that is closest to the athlete's waist on the lower margin of his or her rib cage on the side of the chest that is closest to your knees. You are now in position to find the compression site.

Run your fingers along the rib cage toward the midline. Stop when you find the notch in the lower center of the chest where the ribs meet the breastbone. At this point, your middle finger should be at the notch and your index finger resting against the middle finger. This will place your index finger directly over the lower end of the breastbone.

Place the heel of your other hand over the middle of the breastbone so that the thumb side of this hand touches the index finger, which is positioned at the lower end of the breastbone. Your hand closest to the athlete's head is now directly over the CPR compression site (see Figure 4.7). For children (1-8 years of age) use only one hand to provide compression.

External Chest Compressions

External chest compressions should be delivered in the following manner:

1. Have the athlete properly positioned on his or her back, lying on a hard surface (the ground or floor). Soft surfaces will

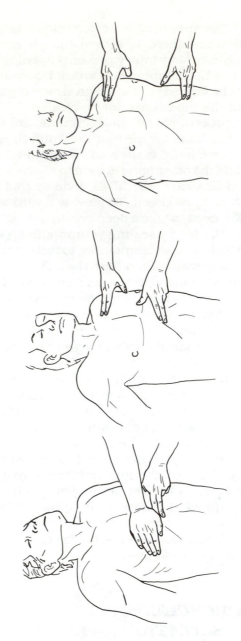

Figure 4.7. Locating the CPR compression site.

make compressions more difficult and less effective.

2. Locate the CPR compression site and have the heel of your hand that is closest to the athlete's head directly on top of this site.

3. If the athlete is a child (1-8 years of age), you will deliver the compressions with the heel of one hand. Two hands are needed when the athlete is an adult. To position the second hand, place the hand you used to find the breastbone notch directly over the top of the first

hand so that their heels are parallel and the fingers point away from your body.

4. Extend both sets of fingers or interlace the fingers of both hands (see Figure 4.8). Regardless of the method you select, you *must* keep the fingers off the athlete's chest to help prevent damaging the breastbone and ribs. If you have arthritis of the hands or if your hand size does not allow you to use either of these methods, you may use the hand that located the breastbone notch to grasp the wrist of the hand that was placed over the compression site.

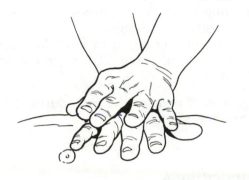

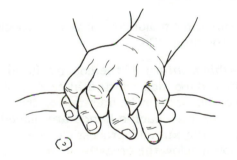

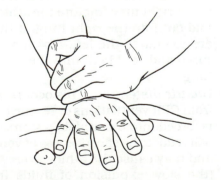

Figure 4.8. Positioning the hands for external chest compressions.

5. Straighten your arms and lock the elbows.
6. Position your shoulders so that they are directly over your hands.

7. Deliver the compressions straight down over the CPR compression site. Make certain that you do not bend your elbows or lift your knees.
8. Apply enough force with each compression so that you depress the adult athlete's breastbone 1½ to 2 inches. The child's breastbone should be depressed 1 to 1½ inches.
9. After compressing the athlete's breastbone, fully release the pressure on the chest. Do *not* lift your hands off the athlete's chest, bend at the elbows, or rock your shoulders from over the top of the CPR compression site. You should lift at the waist so that your shoulders return to their position over the site as shown in Figure 4.9. The time required to release pressure should be equal to that required to compress the breastbone. In other words, the durations for a downstroke and an upstroke are equal.

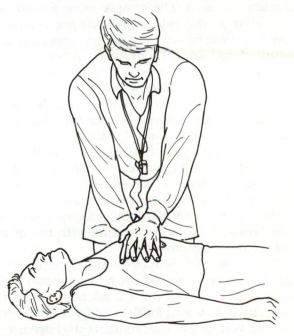

Figure 4.9. Delivering external chest compressions.

Ventilations During CPR

Ventilations can be delivered by the mouth-to-mouth, the mouth-to-nose, or the mouth-to-mouth and nose (for small children) technique. The delivery of ventilations requires you to open the airway by the head-tilt/chin-lift or the jaw-thrust technique. If mouth-to-mouth methods are used, the athlete's nostrils must be pinched shut. Depending on which procedure is used, a tight seal must be formed over the mouth and/or nose. Blow air into the mouth and/or nose until you see the chest rise and you feel resistance to your breaths. The number of breaths you provide at any one time is dependent upon the age of the injured person (see below).

It is important that you establish a regular pattern of breathing for yourself as you perform CPR. If you do not, you may hyperventilate or have trouble delivering ventilations as quickly as possible. Do not try to breathe with each chest compression or hold your breath until a set of compressions is delivered. Breathe as normally as possible during compressions, then take the deep breath necessary for a ventilation.

For CPR performed on the adult athlete, there should be 15 compressions followed by two adequate ventilations. The child will receive five compressions followed by one adequate ventilation. The compressions should be delivered at the rate of 80-100 per minute. Since you will be stopping the compressions for ventilations, only 60 compressions per minute will actually be delivered. The faster rate of 80-100 per minute allows time for ventilations.

To be certain that you are delivering the compressions at the correct rate for an adult athlete, you should count "One-and, two-and, three-and, four-and, five-and . . ." until you have delivered 15 compressions. At the end of the last compression, you should open the athlete's airway and deliver two adequate ventilations. After the ventilations, relocate the CPR compression site and continue with the next set of compressions.

The count and compressions for a child athlete should be "One and two and three and four and five," followed by one adequate breath. Remember to watch for the child's chest to rise so that you do not overventilate and drive air into the stomach.

The CPR Cycle

Perform CPR in the following cycle of activities:

1. After establishing that there is no pulse, find the CPR compression site and position one (child) or both (adult) hands and your shoulders over the compression site.
2. Deliver 5 (child) or 15 (adult) compressions at the rate of 80-100 compressions per minute.
3. Provide one (child) or two (adult) ventilations.
4. After the first minute, stop and check once more for both breathing and carotid pulse.
5. If there is neither breathing nor a pulse, continue CPR with cycles of 5 compressions and one ventilation (child) or 15 compressions and two ventilations (adult).
6. Stop every few minutes to check for breathing and pulse.
7. Give one (child) or two (adult) breaths before beginning CPR after reassessment.

Figure 4.10 reviews the procedures of CPR for the adult victim.

Complications

There are three major complications associated with providing CPR:

- *Athlete injury.* If the coach's hands are placed too high on the athlete's chest, the collarbones may be fractured or dislocated. When the coach's hands are placed too low, the xiphoid process (located at the notch below the breastbone) may cut into the liver. Placement of the hands too far to the right may fracture the athlete's ribs and cut into the right lung. If the hands are too far to the left, ribs may be fractured and could cut into the heart or left lung.
- *Gastric distention.* This occurs when air from CPR ventilations or rescue breathing is forced into the athlete's stomach. This will reduce the effectiveness of ventilations and may cause the athlete to regurgitate (the slow expulsion of fluids from the stomach) or vomit.
- *Regurgitation, or vomiting.* This may occur even when there are no signs of gastric distention. The athlete may breathe in (aspirate) the fluids into his or her lungs.

Functions	
Determine unresponsiveness Position athlete Open airway Look, listen, and feel (3 to 5 seconds for breathing)	
Deliver 2 breaths at 1 to 1 1/2 seconds per ventilation	
Check carotid pulse for 5 to 10 seconds If no pulse, then begin chest compressions	
Compressions 80 to 100/min (15/9 to 11 sec)	
Ventilations 2 ventilations/15 compressions	
Do 4 cycles, then check pulse	
Do periodic assessment of breathing and pulse	

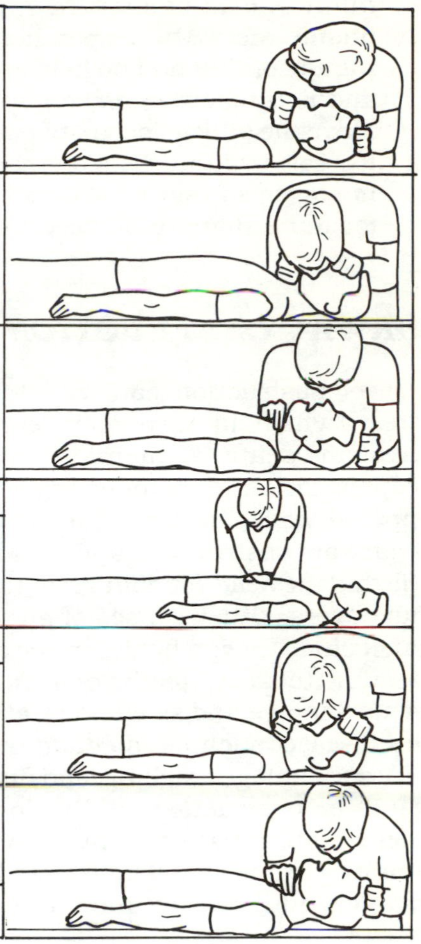

Figure 4.10. One-rescuer CPR.

Proper hand positioning will prevent serious injury to the athlete; however, ribs may fracture or break loose from the breastbone even when CPR is performed correctly. Do *not* stop CPR if this happens but quickly assess your hand positions and the depth of your compressions. Then make the necessary adjustments and continue with CPR.

Do *not* attempt to force air out of the stomach of an athlete who has gastric distention. If you do, he or she may vomit and aspirate the vomitus into the lungs. Simply reposition the athlete's head so that it is properly positioned to receive ventilations and adjust your breath size to deliver enough air to cause the athlete's chest to rise.

When simple regurgitation takes place, the coach is often unaware of the event, so little can be done. If the athlete vomits, clear his or her mouth using the finger-sweep technique (pp. 47-48).

Stopping CPR

Once you have started CPR, you must continue until one of the following occurs:

- You are relieved by someone of equal or greater training
- The athlete regains a carotid pulse (If this happens, provide rescue breathing.)
- The athlete regains spontaneous respirations and a pulse (a rare occurrence)
- You are too exhausted to continue (There are limitations as to what is expected of a person performing CPR, and you should never feel guilty if you reach your physical limitations and help has not arrived.)

Should you find it necessary to interrupt CPR, do not stop the procedure for more than *7 seconds*. Do not interrupt CPR except to

- check for breathing and a pulse after 1 minute of CPR (can be done in 7 seconds);

- check for breathing and a pulse every few minutes (can be done in 7 seconds);
- phone the EMS dispatcher (if after 1 minute of CPR and no help is on the scene and is unlikely to arrive); and
- move the athlete for safety reasons. (When it is safe to do so, the move should be done in stages so that CPR is not interrupted for more than 15-30 seconds at a time.)

AIRWAY OBSTRUCTION

Airway obstruction can lead to respiratory arrest, which in turn may lead to cardiac arrest and death. As mentioned earlier in this chapter, the athlete's tongue may obstruct the upper airway. This is the most common form of airway obstruction and is alleviated by utilizing the head-tilt/chin-lift or the jaw-thrust maneuvers. Other causes of airway obstruction include foreign bodies in the airway, such as gum, tobacco, teeth, or a mouth guard; tissue damage and swelling related to injury; and disease, such as infection or asthma.

Tissue damage, swelling, and disease usually result in obstruction of the lower airway. There is little that you can do for such problems other than to call for immediate EMS assistance and to continue to ventilate the athlete.

The procedures presented in this section deal with foreign-body airway obstruction. The best method of dealing with such obstruction is *prevention*. An athlete should never be allowed to participate in any sport while having food, gum, a toothpick, or a tobacco product in the mouth. As a coach, you must make certain that all mouth guards are of the correct size and fit and that no athlete attempts to use a homemade or a self-repaired device.

Dental appliances can also be sources of an airway obstruction. You must make certain that any athlete who has crowns (caps), decorative inserts, decorative caps, bridges, or dentures (partial or full) has a dental evaluation before being allowed to participate in any event. Partial or full dentures should not be worn for any contact sport or for any sport that may produce falls.

Detecting Obstructions

Airway obstructions can be partial or complete.

Unusual breathing sounds are often associated with partial obstruction. You may hear snoring sounds caused by the tongue obstructing the throat or gurgling due to foreign objects or blood in the airway. You may also notice skin-color changes such as blue or gray skin, lips, tongue, or fingernail beds. Changes in breathing patterns may also indicate a partial obstruction. The athlete may change from normal breathing to very labored breathing then back to normal breathing.

The conscious athlete often will point to his or her mouth or display the universal distress signal of grasping the throat. Ask the athlete if he or she can speak. If the athlete can talk, the obstruction is partial. Next, ask him or her to cough. A strong cough indicates a partial obstruction with adequate air exchange. Keep encouraging the athlete to cough. This will usually dislodge the foreign object. Do *not* interfere with an athlete's effort to cough.

The conscious athlete with a complete airway obstruction will not be able to talk or cough. Almost always, the athlete will display the distress signal for choking. The unconscious athlete with a complete airway obstruction will not display rhythmic chest movements or air exchange at the mouth and nose. This can be quickly detected by the look-listen-feel method.

Correcting Foreign-Object Obstructions

Have the conscious athlete with a partial obstruction cough. Do not take any other action as long as he or she is able to cough forcefully. If the athlete is unable to cough but is still responsive, open the airway in case the tongue is causing the obstruction.

Do *not* slap the athlete on the back. This technique is recommended only for infants, and its use on children and adults may worsen the obstruction. If the obstruction is complete or if the athlete has a partial obstruction but is unable to produce a forceful cough, apply the maneuvers explained in this chapter to clear foreign-object airway obstructions.

Manual Thrusts—The Heimlich Maneuver

The rescuer can apply thrusts to the athlete's abdomen or chest using the hands. These thrusts must be done rapidly to dislodge a foreign object from the airway.

Abdominal Thrusts. If the athlete is conscious and is standing or sitting, stand directly behind him or her and wrap your arms under the armpits and around the waist. Make a fist and place the thumb side of the fist against the athlete's midline, that is, between the rib cage and the waist (see Figure 4.11). Avoid a placement that is too high and that brings you in contact with the lower breastbone (xiphoid process). Use your free hand to grasp the fist and apply six to ten inward thrusts upward toward the athlete's diaphragm.

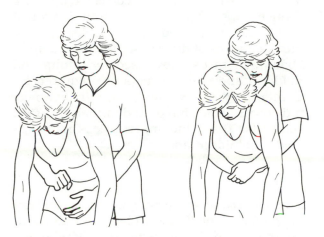

Figure 4.11. The Heimlich Maneuver—rapidly deliver 6 to 10 abdominal thrusts.

If the athlete is unconscious or is unable to sit or stand, place him or her on the back and kneel at the side at hip level. If the athlete is large, you may be able to deliver more effective thrusts if you straddle him or her at the hips. Place the heel of one hand at the athlete's abdominal midline, just above the navel, but not on the rib cage and breastbone. Place your free hand over the top of this hand, position your shoulders over the abdomen, and lock your elbows. Rapidly deliver six to ten abdominal thrusts inward and upward toward the diaphragm.

> **WARNING:**
> Abdominal thrusts should not be delivered to athletes who have abdominal injuries or are pregnant, or to infants.

Chest Thrusts. This method is used for infants or for athletes who have abdominal injuries, or are pregnant. It is also useful when the athlete is too large for you to wrap your arms around his or her waist. If the adult athlete is conscious and is standing or sitting, stand behind him or her and slip your arms under the armpits so that you encircle the chest. Place a fist at the midline of the athlete's breastbone, about two or three finger-widths above the xiphoid process (this is the same as the CPR compression site). Use your free hand to grasp this fist and deliver six to ten thrusts to the chest (use only four thrusts for infants). These thrusts should be pulled directly toward you. Do not pull up or off to the side.

If the adult athlete is unconscious or is unable to sit or stand, place him or her on the back and assume the same position used to deliver external chest compressions during CPR. The hands should be in the same position as in CPR, with the fingers interlocked. Your shoulders should be directly over the compression site and your elbows locked as you rapidly deliver six to ten downward thrusts (use only four thrusts for infants).

If the athlete is a child, use one hand to deliver the compressions. This is done most effectively when the child is lying on his or her back and you are kneeling at the child's feet. If practical, the child can be placed on a table, and you can stand at his or her feet.

Finger Sweeps

> **WARNING:**
> This procedure is recommended for use on unconscious athletes only. Performing this procedure on a conscious person may cause vomiting.

A dislodged or partially dislodged object can be removed by using your fingers to clear the athlete's mouth. Special care must be exercised so that the object is not pushed down the throat, and even more care is needed if the athlete is a child. *Do not perform blind finger sweeps on a child or infant.* You must open the child's mouth and see the object before trying to grasp it or sweep it clear of the airway and mouth.

Tongue-Jaw Lift. The mouth and airway of an unconscious athlete who has an airway obstruction can be opened by using the tongue-jaw lift procedure. Insert your thumb into the athlete's mouth so that you can grasp the tongue and lower jaw between your thumb and fingers, then lift the lower jaw and tongue. This will often move the tongue away from the obstruction. Insert the index finger of your free hand into the athlete's mouth and slide this finger along the inside of the cheek to the base of the tongue. You can use the index finger as a hook to dislodge the obstruction and sweep it forward in the mouth for removal. In some cases you may need to push the object against the opposite side of the throat to lift and sweep it forward, but great care must be taken to avoid pushing the object down the athlete's throat.

Stay alert if you place your fingers in the athlete's mouth. Even the unconscious athlete can suddenly regain consciousness, and you could be severely bitten.

Crossed-Finger Technique. If the unconscious athlete's mouth will not open easily, you can use the crossed-finger technique (see Figure 4.12). Place one hand on the athlete's forehead to stabilize the head. Cross the thumb under the index finger of your free hand. Place your thumb against the athlete's lower lip and your index finger against the upper teeth, then uncross your thumb and finger to force the mouth open. After opening the athlete's mouth, hold the lower jaw so that his or her mouth cannot close. Once the mouth is opened, take your hand from the forehead and use the index finger of this hand to perform finger sweeps to clear the mouth.

Combined Procedures

When an obstruction is not corrected by using a single standard procedure, a combination of procedures can be applied to increase the rescuer's chances of dislodging the obstruction. Abdominal thrusts are used for adults and children, and chest thrusts are required for infants, pregnant women, large individuals, and those who have abdominal injuries. Remember that blind finger sweeps cannot be used on children and infants.

Conscious Athlete

If there is a complete airway obstruction or poor air exchange or if the athlete's condition is declining, you should deliver 6 to 10 abdominal thrusts (adult or child) in rapid succession. If the athlete's airway remains obstructed, you should repeat the sets of thrusts until the airway is clear or the athlete loses consciousness. If the airway does not clear immediately, have someone alert the EMS system.

Athlete Loses Consciousness

If you are trying to clear the athlete's airway and he or she becomes unconscious, protect the athlete from injury and position him or her on the back. Make certain that someone calls for an EMS response as you use the tongue-jaw lift to open the athlete's mouth. Perform finger sweeps, open the athlete's airway, and attempt to deliver two adequate breaths. If this fails, perform six to ten abdominal thrusts in rapid succession. If the airway remains obstructed, check the mouth for foreign bodies and attempt finger sweeps. Next, open the airway and attempt to ventilate the athlete. If this fails, begin the following sequence and continue until the airway is clear:

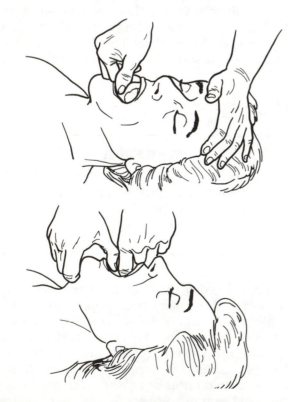

Figure 4.12 The crossed-finger technique can be used to open the unconscious athlete's mouth.

1. Manual thrusts
2. Finger sweeps
3. Ventilations

Continue your attempts to clear the airway. Even a partially dislodged object will allow ventilations to be delivered. With time, the muscles of the lower jaw and the upper airway will relax, thus improving the chances of clearing the airway.

Unconscious Athlete

If the athlete is unconscious when you arrive, establish unresponsiveness, properly position him or her on the back, and open the airway. If the athlete is not breathing, attempt to provide two adequate ventilations. If this fails, reposition the athlete's head and reattempt the ventilations. Should the airway remain obstructed, have someone alert the EMS system while you deliver six to ten abdominal thrusts. If these manual thrusts fail to clear the airway, attempt to ventilate the athlete and repeat the sequence of manual thrusts, finger sweeps, and attempts to ventilate. Continue your efforts until the airway is clear enough to allow for successful rescue breathing.

SUMMARY AND RECOMMENDATIONS

The procedures in basic life support must be learned step by step if they are to be applied properly to save an athlete's life. There are no short cuts with these techniques. As a coach you should be certified in these procedures by the American Heart Association or the American Red Cross and be recertified as recommended by these organizations.

1. To carry out basic life support properly, you must be able to establish unresponsiveness, position the athlete, open the airway (head-tilt/chin-lift or jaw-thrust procedures), determine breathlessness (look-listen-feel method), and deliver adequate mouth-to-mouth or mouth-to-nose ventilations.
2. Ventilations should last 1-1.5 seconds each, with the athlete's chest being watched to ensure proper delivery.
3. During rescue breathing, the adult should receive one breath every 5 seconds. The child should be given one breath every 4 seconds.
4. Performing CPR requires that you establish the lack of pulse (carotid pulse check), position the athlete, find the CPR compression site, properly place your hands, and deliver smooth chest compressions at a rate of 80-100 per minute.
5. The adult's chest is compressed 1½ to 2 inches 15 times, followed by two ventilations. Compression for the child should be 1 to 1½ inches, repeated 5 times, followed by one adequate breath.
6. These compression and ventilation cycles are repeated until you are relieved, function is restored, or fatigue forces you to discontinue CPR.
7. You must know how to clear an obstructed airway using manual thrusts, finger sweeps, and ventilations. Abdominal thrusts are to be used for both children and adults.
8. Blind finger sweeps cannot be used if the athlete is under 8 years of age.

Chapter 5
Bleeding and Shock

Coaches will most likely face very few life-threatening injuries; however, when they do occur, they often involve bleeding or the development of shock. Many mild or moderate injuries can quickly become severe if either of these two problems is not cared for properly. It is essential that you know how to handle both emergencies.

THE CONTROL OF BLEEDING

As blood circulates, it carries oxygen and nutrients to the body's tissues and assists in temperature regulation. It also picks up and transports carbon dioxide and other waste products that will be eliminated from the body and moves hormones and other key chemicals from one place in the body to another. Any significant loss of blood can quickly disrupt or lower the efficiency of these essential functions and put the person in critical condition.

Blood circulates through three types of blood vessels. Blood leaving the heart is carried through the *arteries*. The pressure in these vessels is at a higher level than it is in the other vessels of the circulatory system. Blood returns to the heart through the *veins*. The pressure in these vessels is significantly lower than that in the arteries. Between arteries and veins are the *capillaries*, where exchange between the blood and the tissues takes place. The blood moves through the capillaries in a smooth, constant flow. This process is called *perfusion* and is essential to life. Any major loss of blood can cause perfusion to fail, so the control of bleeding must be a primary concern.

Classifying Bleeding

It is often useful to classify the type of bleeding to be controlled into two systems: by the type of blood vessel and by the location of the bleeding.

Type of Blood Vessel

Bleeding can be classified on the basis of the type of vessel that is losing blood. According to this classification, there are three types of bleeding: arterial, venous, and capillary.

Loss of blood from an artery is always serious and is often profuse (great enough to be life threatening). Bright red blood flows freely from the wound in spurts that occur each time the heart beats. Arteries carry oxygenated blood from the heart to the body.

If a large vein is injured, bleeding may be profuse; however, even then, venous bleeding does not display the spurts seen in arterial bleeding. Instead, the loss is seen as a steady flow, with the blood often appearing to be dark red or maroon. Veins carry deoxygenated blood back to the heart.

Capillary bleeding is the loss of red blood from a capillary bed. The blood is less bright than that seen during arterial bleeding, and the loss takes place slowly, usually oozing from the wound. Capillary bleeding is the least serious form of bleeding but should be controlled, and steps should be taken to reduce contamination.

Location of the Bleeding

Bleeding may also be classified on the basis of where in the body the bleeding is taking place.

A general system of classification considers bleeding to be internal or external. You will usually not be able to tell what type of blood vessels are involved when the bleeding is internal.

Controlling External Bleeding

External bleeding is detected simply by looking for the loss of blood. The rate of blood loss, its color, and the appearance of the flow (spurting, steady flow, or oozing) is usually obvious.

There are three methods that can be applied to control external bleeding:

- Direct pressure
- Direct pressure and elevation
- Arterial pressure points

Direct Pressure

This is the primary way you should attempt to control bleeding. If bleeding is not profuse, apply pressure by holding a sterile dressing directly over the top of the wound. A clean cloth or handkerchief may be used if no sterile dressing is immediately available. Blood-soaked dressings should not be removed as this could disrupt the clot and restart bleeding. Always place fresh dressings directly over the top of the blood-soaked ones (see Figure 5.1).

If bleeding is profuse, *do not waste time hunting* for a dressing. Place your hand over the top of the wound and apply firm, steady pressure.

> **WARNING:**
> Direct contact with another person's blood may lead to infection. This is especially true if you have cuts, sores, or other breaks in your skin. The greatest risk is hepatitis and other viral diseases. Concern over the transmission of Acquired Immune Deficiency Syndrome, or AIDS, has led many EMS systems to recommend wearing rubber or latex gloves if contact may be made with any injured person's blood or body fluids. For maximum protection against such transmission, all individuals who are called on to render care should have available disposable, sterile gloves and wear them as the circumstance warrants.

In either case, pressure should be applied until the bleeding is controlled (this may take 5 or more minutes). After this is done, a dressing may be added and bandaged in place. Remember, if a dressing was used initially, it should *not* be removed from the wound but

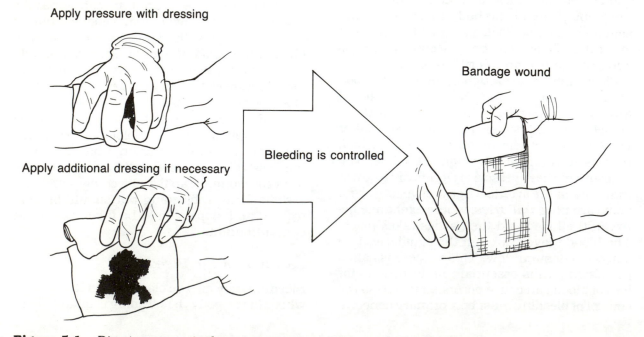

Apply pressure with dressing

Apply additional dressing if necessary

Bleeding is controlled

Bandage wound

Figure 5.1.   Direct pressure is the primary means used to control bleeding.

should be bandaged in place once the bleeding is controlled.

A special form of direct pressure is applying a pressure dressing to control bleeding from an extremity. The pressure dressing can be especially useful if you have additional injuries to care for. However, it is of little use if bleeding is from the armpit, chest, or abdomen and is of no practical use if bleeding involves a large artery or a deep vein. This method should never be used to control bleeding from the neck.

To use a pressure dressing, do the following (see Figure 5.2):

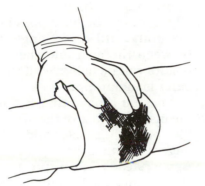

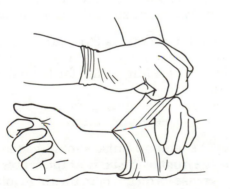

Figure 5.2. A pressure dressing uses a bandage to apply pressure over the top of a bulky dressing.

1. Place gauze pads over top of the wound.
2. Apply and maintain pressure with your hand.
3. Place several handkerchiefs, a sanitary napkin, or a commercial bulky dressing over the gauze pads and immediately apply pressure with your hand.
4. Hold these dressings in place with a self-adherent roller bandage (e.g., Kling), wrap the bandage so that it covers the dressings and the areas above and

below the wound (proximal and distal), and continue to wrap the bandage until enough pressure has been created to control the bleeding.
5. Make certain that you can detect a distal pulse in the injured limb. The correct pressure will control the bleeding without stopping circulation. If there is a loss of distal pulse after the dressing and bandage have been applied, you will have to reduce some of the pressure that has been applied.

For all injuries that involve external bleeding other than mild capillary or simple-cut bleeding, you *must* have someone alert the EMS system dispatcher. Injuries that cause moderate bleeding may be more serious than you can determine. Controlled moderate bleeding may degenerate into profuse bleeding. All cases of profuse bleeding require EMS intervention as soon as possible. Bleeding from the eye, ear, nose, or mouth requires special techniques that will be covered in later chapters on wound care.

Direct Pressure and Elevation

Direct pressure and elevation can be combined to improve the control of bleeding from an extremity. This is recommended when direct pressure alone does not quickly control the bleeding. When the limb is elevated, the effects of gravity will help lower the blood pressure in the injured limb and reduce the flow of blood.

Do *not* use this method if any of the following conditions exist:

- Possible fractures to the extremity, including the pelvis, hip joint, or shoulder joint
- Objects are impaled in the injured extremity
- Possible injuries to the neck or spine

To combine direct pressure and elevation do the following (see Figure 5.3):

1. Apply direct pressure as soon as possible as you would to control most forms of bleeding.
2. Maintain this pressure while elevating the injured limb or the affected part of the limb to a point where the wound is above the level of the heart (e.g., if the

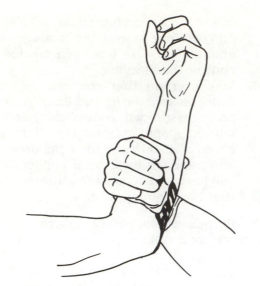

Figure 5.3. Direct pressure and elevation can be combined to control bleeding from an extremity.

bleeding is from the forearm, it is necessary to elevate only the forearm, not the entire arm).

3. Continue to hold the limb in its elevated position and apply pressure to the wound site until bleeding is controlled.

Arterial Pressure Points

Where an artery lies close to the body surface and is directly over the top of a bone, pressure may be applied to reduce or stop the flow of blood. Arterial pressure points should be used only after direct pressure or direct pressure and elevation have failed to control the bleeding adequately. If there are possible fractures to a limb, applying pressure-point techniques may cause more bleeding if the broken bones cut through soft tissues and blood vessels.

There are 11 arterial pressure-point sites on each side of the body. Only two sites—one in the thigh and one in the upper arm—are of use in field emergency care: The brachial artery pressure point is used to control profuse bleeding from the arm, and the femoral artery pressure point is used to control bleeding from the leg.

If your attempts to control bleeding from the arm using direct pressure and direct pressure and elevation fail, take the following steps (see Figure 5.4):

1. Maintain direct pressure over the wound site and move the injured athlete's

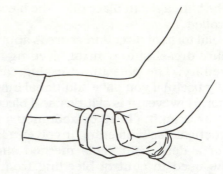

Figure 5.4. The brachial pressure-point technique can control bleeding from the arm.

upper limb so that it extends out laterally from the body. If possible, extend the limb until a 90° angle is formed between the arm and the chest. Best results will be achieved if the athlete's palm is facing up.

2. Locate the groove that is found along the inside surface of the arm just below the biceps muscle and place your fingers in this groove.
3. Apply steady, firm pressure in the groove until the bleeding stops. If pressure is applied correctly, there will be no radial pulse in the injured limb.

Because of the complex circulation pattern in the arm, this technique is not very effective in controlling bleeding at the far (distal) end of the arm.

To control bleeding from the leg, follow these steps (see Figure 5.5):

1. The femoral pulse should be found on the front of the body at the center of the crease formed where the thigh joins the trunk.
2. Apply steady, firm pressure at this site using the heel of your hand. The muscles of the thigh will offer resistance to your attempts to compress the femoral artery, so you will need to apply much more pressure than that required for the brachial pressure point. You must keep your arm straight over the top of the femoral pressure-point site and use your body weight to apply the necessary pressure to control bleeding.

Because of the complex circulatory pattern in the leg, this technique is not very effective when bleeding is from the distal end of the leg.

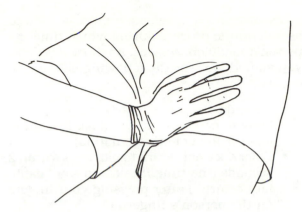

Figure 5.5. The femoral pressure-point technique can control bleeding from the leg.

Caring for Internal Bleeding

Internal bleeding may be no more than a bruise, or it could be a life-threatening problem. Some forms of internal bleeding are difficult to detect and require special tests at a medical center. Most often, you will be able to suspect internal bleeding when you consider the nature of an injury and certain symptoms and signs. You must assume that serious internal bleeding is occurring whenever you detect the following:

- A possible fracture to the pelvis
- A possible fracture to the thigh
- A possible fracture to the upper arm
- Wounds that have penetrated the chest, abdomen, or pelvis
- A large bruise on the neck
- A possible skull fracture or penetrating wounds to the head
- A hardness or spasm of the abdominal muscles or abdominal tenderness
- Large bruises on the chest or indications of possible multiple rib fractures
- Blood, clear fluids, or bloody fluids in the ear or nose
- The athlete coughing up or vomiting blood
- Bleeding from the rectum or vagina
- The athlete reporting blood in his or her urine

If the athlete is injured and has serious internal bleeding, some of the symptoms and signs of shock (covered later in this chapter) will probably be present. Remember that none of these symptoms and signs may be present at the early stages of internal bleeding. If the

mechanism of injury or the nature of the injury can be associated with internal bleeding, assume that internal bleeding is occurring.

Effective field care for internal bleeding requires equipment and techniques that are not available to you. When you suspect internal bleeding, you should take the following action:

1. Have someone alert the EMS system dispatcher.
2. Provide an open airway and monitor the athlete's pulse.
3. Keep the athlete at rest and provide emotional support.
4. Treat for shock (see pp. 56-57).
5. Loosen restrictive clothing.
6. Refrain from giving the athlete anything by mouth and be prepared for vomiting.
7. Splint fractures when appropriate.
8. Constantly monitor the athlete until the EMS system can respond.

SHOCK

One of the most serious complications of any injury or illness is the development of shock. *Trauma* is a term used to mean injury and the conditions brought about by the injury. The injury can be due to an accident, an act of aggression, or the result of an illness. The body's reaction to trauma is *shock*. In most cases, shock develops because the cardiovascular system fails to supply an adequate supply of blood to all the body's vital tissues. When shock occurs, perfusion (smooth flow of the blood through the capillaries) has failed.

An example of shock is the body's reaction to a rapid loss of blood. As blood is being lost, the heart begins to beat faster in an effort to continue the circulation of blood to the body's vital organs. This causes a greater loss of blood, which then forces the heart to beat even more rapidly. The process may continue until the person dies.

If shock is present, then at least one of four things has occurred:

- The heart has failed as a pump and can no longer pump an adequate supply of blood (as with a heart attack)
- Blood vessels have dilated (increased in diameter) to a point where the circulatory system's volume is too large to be filled

by the blood that is available (as when the spine is injured and nerves controlling blood-vessel diameter can no longer function)
• There is not enough fluid available for circulation (as the result of profuse bleeding)
• Breathing problems have resulted in insufficient amounts of oxygen being circulated through the body

Many factors can cause shock to develop. Coaches may see shock induced by blood loss, spinal or nerve damage that causes the control over blood-vessel diameter to be lost, or an extreme allergic reaction that rapidly affects the heart and the diameter of the blood vessels. Some people go into shock from complications associated with fractures and other less serious injuries as well. So, it is important that you learn to handle shock effectively.

Symptoms and Signs of Shock

Shock may develop slowly or rapidly. Sometimes the athlete may show no signs during the early stages, or the signs detected may be mild as the body tries to compensate for the shock. All the symptoms and signs of shock will not usually be present at once.

Before learning how the symptoms and signs of shock occur as shock develops, you should consider all the possible symptoms and signs as they might be detected during the assessment.

The symptoms of shock may include these characteristics:

• Restlessness, anxiety, fear, irritability, or aggressiveness
• Nausea (with or without vomiting)
• Weakness
• Thirst
• Dizziness

The signs of shock may include the following:

• Restlessness
• Changes in the state of awareness
• Shallow and rapid breathing
• Rapid and weak pulse
• Pale, cool, and clammy skin
• Blue or gray coloration to the face or color changes at the tongue, lips, or nail beds
• Dilated pupils and dull eyes

Because shock develops, it must be viewed as a *dynamic* process during which time the person's condition worsens. As shock develops, you should look for the following changes to occur:

• A rapid pulse rate (an early attempt by the body to compensate for blood loss, fluid loss, or inefficient circulation)
• Color does not return to nail beds within 2 seconds (the time it takes to say "capillary return") after pressing your fingers on the person's fingernail
• A rapid breathing rate
• Restlessness, anxiety, fear, or irritability (or the person becoming combative)
• Skin-color changes and the skin feeling cool to the touch
• The person complains of thirst, nausea, and/or weakness
• The pulse becomes rapid and weak and breathing is weak and labored
• The person becomes disoriented, complains of being sleepy, or becomes unconscious
• Respiratory, then cardiac, arrest develops

The bodies of athletes under the age of 35 and especially those of children and adolescents may be able to compensate and hold off the development of shock at times. The compensation does not last for long, and once it is lost the individual's condition declines very rapidly. Always assume that shock is developing when the athlete experiences moderate to severe bleeding, possible spinal injury, major injuries (e.g., a fractured femur), multiple injuries, or unconsciousness.

Care for Shock

The basic care for shock includes the following (see Figure 5.6):

1. Have someone alert the EMS system dispatcher.
2. Keep the athlete at rest, lying down.
3. Make certain that there is an open airway.
4. Control all serious external bleeding.
5. Splint major fractures.
6. Cover the athlete as soon as possible. When it is practical to do so, place one blanket under and one blanket over the

injured athlete, keeping the head uncovered. Do *not* allow the athlete to overheat as this will aggravate his or her condition.

7. Properly position the injured athlete. If there are no indications of spinal, pelvic, or lower-extremity injuries, place the athlete flat on his or her back, elevating the legs 8-10 inches. If this is not possible because of injuries, keep the athlete lying flat. For cases involving shock and respiratory problems where the airway is clear, it is acceptable to position the conscious athlete in a semiseated position (slightly raise the chest, shoulders, neck, and head). This can be done only if there is no possibility of spinal, neck, chest, or abdominal injuries.

8. Do *not* give the athlete anything by mouth. Be prepared for vomiting.

9. Provide emotional support to the athlete.

10. Assess pulse and respirations at least once every 5 minutes. Wait with the athlete until medical assistance arrives.

Anaphylactic Shock

Anaphylactic shock is "allergy shock" and develops when someone has an extreme reaction to a substance to which he or she is allergic (an allergen). No matter how mild the initial stages may appear, this must be considered to be a true emergency that requires a physician's care or EMS intervention as soon as possible. It is not possible to determine whether the athlete's body will correct itself, remain stable, or rapidly grow worse and develop a life-threatening condition.

Anaphylactic shock may be brought about by several allergens:

- Inhaled substances such as dust and pollens
- Insect bites and stings
- Foods and spices
- Inhaled chemicals or skin contact with certain chemicals
- Medications (e.g., penicillin)

The symptoms and signs of anaphylactic shock include any or all of the following (see Figure 5.7):

- Restlessness
- Difficult breathing (wheezing sometimes occurs)
- Rapid, weak pulse
- Itching or burning skin
- Development of hives
- Swelling at the face and tongue
- Blue coloration to the tongue and lips
- Fainting or unconsciousness

The care provided for an athlete developing anaphylactic shock is the same as the care you would render for any type of shock. If the shock is related to an insect sting, remove the stinger and venom sack. This can usually be done by scraping away the stinger with a plastic credit card. Make certain that the EMS system is responding and knows that the athlete may be developing anaphylactic shock.

Some people who are allergic to bee stings or who have other severe allergy problems carry medications to be taken during an emergency. You may assist the person in taking his or her medications; however, if the person cannot actually take the medicine by him- or herself, you may not inject or otherwise give him or her the medication unless the laws in your

Ensure open airway and breathing
Elevate uninjured lower extremities
Prevent loss of body heat
Give nothing by mouth

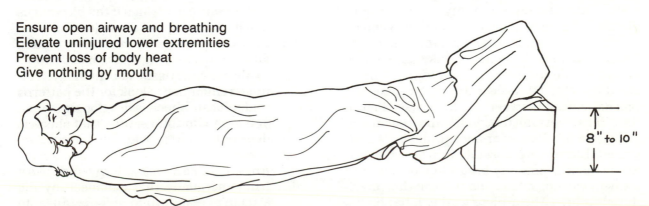

Figure 5.6. Providing care for the athlete who is developing shock.

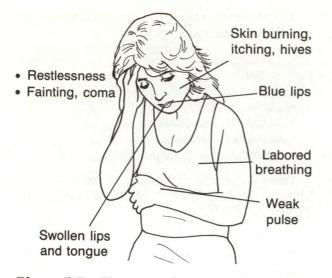

- Restlessness
- Fainting, coma

Skin burning, itching, hives

Blue lips

Labored breathing

Weak pulse

Swollen lips and tongue

Figure 5.7. The signs of anaphylactic shock.

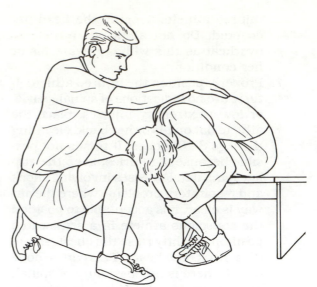

Figure 5.8. Positioning an athlete to prevent fainting.

state allow you to do so. Seek professional legal advice concerning the laws in your state.

Fainting

Fainting is a mild, self-correcting form of shock that is usually brought on by fear, stress, or an emotional crisis. It also may be a warning of more serious problems such as fluid loss or undetected medical problems. Do *not* consider fainting to be a minor problem, especially if there is no obvious emotional problem causing the episode. Rest the athlete while having a nurse, doctor, or medical assistant monitor his or her blood pressure. Also be sure to check for any injuries that may have been sustained during the fall. Insist that the athlete see a doctor as soon as possible. Until the athlete is seen by a physician, he or she should not participate in any athletic event, operate machinery, or drive a motor vehicle.

When you suspect that a person is about to faint, you may be able to take preventive action or offer protection from injury if he or she does faint. Seat the uninjured athlete and place the head between the knees (see Figure 5.8). Make certain that you can prevent the athlete from falling over once he or she is positioned. If there are possible injuries, the athlete is having difficulty breathing, or there are known heart problems, do *not* use this procedure but have the athlete lie down flat on his or her back.

SUMMARY AND RECOMMENDATIONS

Most problems that involve bleeding can be cared for easily. The more serious forms of bleeding require a quick assessment and immediate action.

Keep the following information in mind:

1. Direct pressure is the primary means used to control external bleeding.
2. Internal bleeding must be assumed if the mechanism of injury, the type of injury, and the patient assessment indicate that it is a possibility. The symptoms and signs of shock are usually associated with serious internal bleeding. As a result, you should provide care in the same manner as you would for shock, use pressure dressings if the bleeding is in a limb, and splint all major fractures.
3. Shock develops as the circulatory system fails to provide an adequate blood supply to all the vital tissues of the body. You must remember to look for the patterns that indicate shock is developing. When you are in doubt, assume that shock is developing and provide the appropriate care.
4. Anaphylactic shock (allergy shock) is a true emergency that is caused by the athlete's reaction to a substance to which he or she is extremely allergic.

This type of shock requires a physician or EMS intervention as soon as possible. While waiting for the physician or EMS personnel to arrive, treat the athlete for shock.

5. Fainting is a mild, self-correcting form of shock usually caused by an emotional reaction. Do *not* consider fainting to be of minor importance. The athlete should be seen by a physician.

Chapter 6

Soft-Tissue Injuries— Principles of Wound Care

The body's soft tissues are the skin, blood vessels, nerves, muscles, tendons, ligaments, glands, and linings and coverings of the organs. The hard tissues are the bones, teeth, and cartilage.

Most sport-related soft-tissue wounds are confined to the skin, the body's largest organ in terms of size. The skin protects the body, acting as a barrier to disease-causing organisms and keeping underlying structures from direct contact with the environment. Additional protection is provided in the form of shock absorption as the skin cushions the shock of blows with the help of the underlying layers of fat.

The skin is also involved with temperature regulation, water balance, and excretion. It allows excess heat to radiate from its blood vessels, provides insulation with its fats, and the sweat glands in the skin produce perspiration to cool the body through evaporation. The skin's most important water-balance function is to prevent the direct loss or gain of water from the environment. Since the skin is highly involved with the release of salts, carbon dioxide, and excess water through the sweat glands and pores, it must be considered to be a major organ of excretion.

Some sensory perception is also carried out in the skin. Specialized nerve endings in the

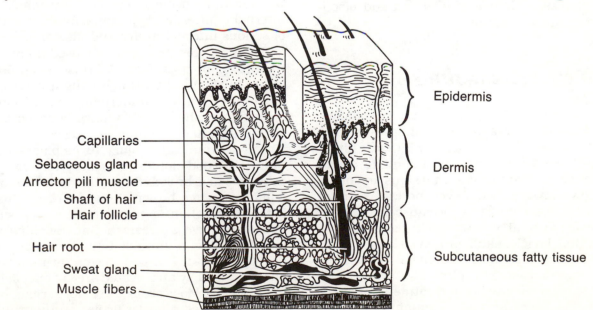

Capillaries

Sebaceous gland

Arrector pili muscle

Shaft of hair

Hair follicle

Hair root

Sweat gland

Muscle fibers

Epidermis

Dermis

Subcutaneous fatty tissue

Figure 6.1.   The structures of the skin.

skin act as receptors for heat, cold, pain, pressure, and touch.

There are two main layers to the skin: the epidermis and the dermis. A third layer, the subcutaneous layers, lies beneath the dermis and is often discussed in conjunction with the skin (see Figure 6.1).

The *epidermis*, or surface layer, is free of blood vessels and nerves. Except for thermal burns, serious sunburn, and exposure to excessive cold, injuries to the epidermis are seldom difficult to care for.

Immediately below the epidermis lies the second layer, the *dermis*. Unlike the epidermis, this skin layer contains blood vessels and nerves and is rich with capillaries and nerve endings. When the dermis is injured, bleeding and pain can range from minor and mild to profuse and intense. Some degree of swelling occurs at and around the injury site, and infection is always a possibility. Since the circulatory system has been opened, bloodstream infection and the spread of infection may occur.

The dermis contains many specialized structures, including sweat glands, sebaceous (oil) glands, hair follicles and roots, and sensory nerve receptors. These structures are so numerous that the damage caused by most wounds does not significantly reduce their functions.

The *subcutaneous* layers are fat and soft tissues found below the dermis. Injury to these layers produces pain, bleeding, swelling, and an increased chance of infection and bloodstream contamination.

SOFT-TISSUE INJURIES

The structures that make up the body's systems—the organs and glands—are composed of soft tissues. Most injuries to these structures are minor and difficult to detect because there are no external signs and onset is slow. However, whenever there are signs of organ or gland injury or the cause of an injury (a severe forceful blow or a fractured bone such as a rib, clavicle, skull, or pelvis) leads you to believe that there may be damage to the internal organs, care by a physician is required. There is no effective field treatment for these injuries. Never accept statements such as, "Don't worry about it. He probably bruised his

kidney. Give him a cold pack." Doctors do not make guesses about internal injuries but will want to examine the patient and run the necessary tests. The athlete with a possible internal organ injury *must* see a physician. If you suspect internal injuries, treat the athlete for shock and alert the EMS system of your suspicion.

CLOSED WOUNDS

Many soft-tissue injuries are classified as closed wounds. With the exception of bruises, most closed wounds can be given little specialized care in the field. A physician's intervention is usually required to assess the nature of the injury properly and to select the necessary care procedures.

A closed wound has no opening between the injury site and the outside environment. It is an internal injury even when it occurs deep within the skin and is visible from the outside. Most closed injuries are caused by the impact of a blunt object or a minor fall. The typical sport-related closed injury is the simple bruise; however, more serious or life-threatening problems can occur. Closed soft-tissue injuries include the damage done to blood vessels, nerves, muscles, and organs when bones are fractured and the rupture of internal organs from severe impacts and serious falls. As a coach, you must consider the mechanism of injury (the way the injury occurred) and the possibility of internal injuries, and you must look for signs of serious internal injury and bleeding.

The most common form of closed injury is the bruise, or *contusion*. A bruise is a crush injury in which soft tissue is caught between the impact and the underlying bone. Blood from the crushed vessels flows between tissues to produce swelling and discoloration. The area around the injury turns black-and-blue as a blood clot forms at the site. Slowly, as the blood is broken down, the discoloration will change to a brownish-yellow color. Just before absorption is complete, the area will appear to have a greenish tint. Swelling is usually evident immediately, but may be delayed for a day or two. Severe bruises are characterized by an elevated area of purplish-red coloring. Most bruises are not serious injuries; however, a larger bruise on the trunk may be a sign of serious internal injury and bleeding. When you find a large bruise, look for possible fractures and other injuries.

Repeated blows to the same site may result in the formation of bone within the muscle tissue (myositis ossificans). This complication is sometimes seen in football players. Thigh pads and upper arm pads can be worn to prevent this injury problem.

CLOSED-WOUND CARE

The severity of an injury must be assessed. The most important factor is the mechanism of injury. When an athlete falls off a high piece of gymnastic apparatus or collides strongly with a piece of apparatus, the only immediate sign of injury may be a small bruise. Blows from bats, sticks, and clubs or with baseballs, lacrosse balls, and golf balls may produce nothing more than a bruise. Each of these accidents can often produce other more serious injuries, so be sure to check for the symptoms and signs of other possible injuries.

You can care for a mild bruise, in which muscle spasms are absent or momentary, stiffness is absent or minor, and little force was involved in causing the injury. There usually is pain at the site, but a point-tenderness test should not cause excessive pain. There is no loss of function associated with mild bruises.

If the athlete has moderate to severe pain, point tenderness, stiffness, loss of function, or muscle spasms that last for several minutes or longer, check for other injuries, immobilize the injured part (see chapter 10), and be sure the athlete receives medical attention. The same procedures apply if swelling and discoloration occur rapidly. Such bruises may involve the underlying bone. In some cases, it is difficult to differentiate between a serious bruise and a nondisplaced fracture without an X ray.

Small, mild bruises usually do not require any special care. However, a bruise that interferes with function should be treated by the "RICE" method:

R = **Rest** (to prevent additional injury and promote healing)

I = **Ice** (to control swelling by constricting blood vessels in the injured area and to reduce pain)

C = **Compression** (to decrease underlying blood flow and to control swelling)

E = **Elevation** (to enable gravity to help with the return of blood to the heart from the injury site and to decrease blood pressure)

The RICE method should not be used if the athlete has a history of circulatory disease or Raynaud's Syndrome (spasms in the arteries of the extremities that reduce circulation) or if the injured part has been previously frostbitten. For those with Raynaud's Syndrome, exposure to cold restricts circulation to the fingers and toes. The digits turn white and become uncomfortably cold. This condition, as well as a history of circulatory problems, should appear in the athlete's medical history. If no fracture is suspected, elevate the body part to help control swelling.

The RICE method should not be employed if

- there are symptoms and signs of fracture or discoloration (Never elevate a limb that may be fractured until it has been properly splinted.);
- there are serious open wounds at or near the bruise site or anywhere on the same limb;
- the injury is to the scalp, face, or neck (Cold can be applied, but there should be no compression.); and
- the athlete will remain exposed to a cold environment.

The first element of the RICE method is rest. The critical question is, How long should an injured athlete rest if the injury is no more than a bruise? The answer depends on the severity of the bruise and its location. If the bruise is minor and if there is no loss of function or range of motion, rest is not important. However, if the bruise produces discomfort that interferes with enjoying the sport and with performance, the athlete should be allowed to rest until the discomfort goes away and function returns to normal. If the bruise is on the sole of the foot, palm of the hand, or some other area that could be aggravated by participation, the athlete needs to rest from activity until the bruise has healed to prevent reinjury. Most bruises require no more than 1-3 days of rest; however, severe bruises may take longer to heal and require protective padding when the athlete returns to activity.

The location and extent of the bruise, as well as the presence of impaired function, determine the amount of time an athlete may be out of activity. For example, bruises to the anterior thigh, hip, neck, or low back may require a longer rest period because of the occurrence of protective muscle spasms, formation of hematomas, inability to function or move normally, and involvement of underlying organs (e.g., kidneys). Recurrent injury at these sites is more likely but may not be as severe. Also, symptoms and signs of a more serious injury, such as kidney damage following a blow to the low back, may be delayed.

The next step is to apply a cold pack with pressure to the injury site to reduce pain and swelling (see Figure 6.2). The pack or ice bag should be wrapped in a wet towel or in other cloth material. In an extremely cold environment, use a dry towel to wrap the cold pack. This will help prevent frostbite. If the purpose of the pack is to reduce the pain of a small bruise, it can be held in place by hand or secured with a cravat (a strip of cloth folded to a width that will extend beyond the edges of the pack); otherwise, compression must be applied.

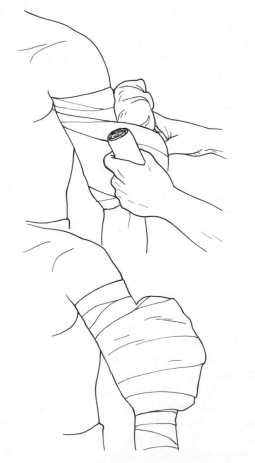

Figure 6.2. A cold pack can help reduce pain and swelling.

You can apply compression with a cravat, but do not allow the cloth to bind the tissues at its edges. Remember to tie the knot over the ice pack and not against the athlete's skin. Elastic bandages are usually used, but be careful not to apply the bandage too tightly as this will restrict circulation. If the elastic bandage is too tight, the athlete will complain of discomfort, a tingling sensation, or the feeling of numbness. Although these sensations are also stages of reaction to ice, there may be swelling below the level of the bandage or the tissue may turn bluish. It is always wise to check for a distal pulse after applying compression.

The cold pack should be applied for no more than 20-30 minutes. After removing the pack, keep the affected part compressed with an elastic bandage and elevated. Wait 90 minutes before reapplying a cold pack. The procedure can be repeated two or three times a day for the next 48-72 hours. If the signs or symptoms worsen or if pain and swelling have not improved, the athlete *must* see a physician.

During cold therapy you can expect the following progression of reactions to cold:

- Cold
- Burning
- Tingling
- Aching
- Numbness

Alert your athletes to these stages and be aware of them yourself. Failure to leave ice in place throughout these stages will result in ineffective cold therapy.

OPEN WOUNDS

The skin is damaged in an open-wound injury. Its surface is usually torn from the outside; however, an open wound is also produced when the skin is torn from the inside by the sharp edges of fractured bone. There are four major types of open injury (see Figure 6.3).

Abrasions

Simple scratches and scrapes to the skin are called *abrasions*. Examples include mat or floor burns, artificial turf (''rug'') burns, and skinned knees and elbows. The injury to the

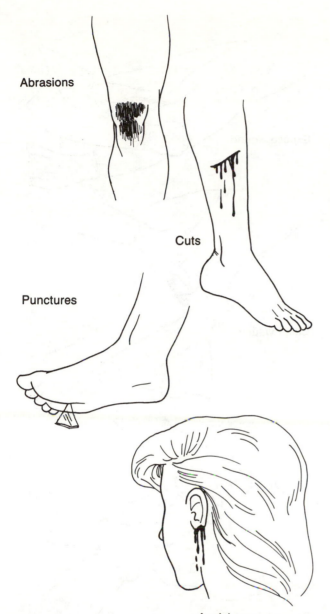

Abrasions

Cuts

Punctures

Avulsions

Figure 6.3.   Types of open wounds.

tissue is not serious, and bleeding often is undetectable, being limited to minor capillary flow. The major concern is contamination or infection.

Cuts

A cut penetrates the skin. Sharp objects produce smooth cuts with straight edges, while rough or dull-edged objects produce jagged cuts. The impact from a blunt object also may produce a jagged cut. Smooth cuts are called

incisions, and jagged cuts are called *lacerations.* The major concerns are bleeding and contamination, which can lead to infection.

Punctures

A puncture wound, most commonly occurring in baseball or track-and-field events, passes through the skin in a straight line. All the tissues in the pathway are damaged. Penetration can be caused by sharp, pointed objects such as spikes, nails, and splinters and can be shallow or deep with blood-vessel damage. If the wound passes through the body (having an entrance and an exit wound), it is called a *perforating wound.* The major concerns with these are bleeding, damage to internal structures, and possible infection. Internal bleeding may be absent or mild.

Avulsions

This type of injury usually involves the skin when a large flap is torn loose or pulled off. The term *avulsion* is used to describe any tissue torn partially or completely from the body. When a tooth is pulled from its socket, it is called an avulsed tooth. The major concerns are bleeding, contamination, and poor tissue healing due to extensive tissue damage. A serious avulsion can lead to disfigurement or loss of use.

OPEN-WOUND CARE

Protect yourself from direct contact with the athlete's blood and body fluids. Use sterile, nonporous, disposable latex or rubber gloves during assessment and care. Remember, you must properly dispose of all contaminated gloves, dressings, and bandages. Disinfect any contaminated surfaces using a solution of 1 part bleach to 10 parts water. Use cleansers containing 2% nonoxynol-9 to wash your hands.

When caring for most open wounds, you should take the following action (see Figure 6.4):

1. *Expose the wound site.* If the mechanism of injury indicates a minor wound

and if bleeding is not profuse, clothing can be removed to give you an un-obstructed view of the wound site. If there is the possibility of a major wound with other injuries, or if bleeding is serious, do not remove clothing in the typical manner as this may worsen existing injuries. Instead, lift or cut away the clothing with bandage shears or a seam cutter.

2. *Clean or clear the wound surface.* Minor scrapes, scratches, and cuts can be cleaned prior to dressing. If the wound is a deep cut, puncture wound, or avulsion, do not attempt to clean the wound or remove debris from inside it. For these types of injury, remove foreign debris from the surface. A physician must cleanse the wound.
3. *Control bleeding.* If bleeding is profuse, the control of blood loss is the first priority. To control bleeding, use the methods described in chapter 5.
4. *Apply a dressing.* Use a sterile dressing that covers the wound completely. If the wound is a minor one, simply apply a bandaid.
5. *Bandage the dressing.*
6. *Reassure the athlete.* Some people, especially young children, need reassurance during and immediately after care.

If there is moderate soft-tissue injury to an extremity, elevate the limb. Do not do this prior to splinting if there are any possible fractures or dislocations.

When the injury is serious or there is profuse bleeding, make certain that the EMS system has been activated or that required health care personnel are alerted. Attempt to control the bleeding while you keep the athlete lying still to reduce circulation. Reassure the athlete and treat for shock. If an extremity is injured but is free of possible fractures or dislocations, it may be helpful to immobilize it to aid in the control of bleeding.

Wound Cleaning

You can clean the surface of scratches, scrapes, and small, shallow cuts that are free of significant bleeding. Wash the surface with mild soap and water. Do not use antibacterial or deodorant soaps to cleanse the wound because

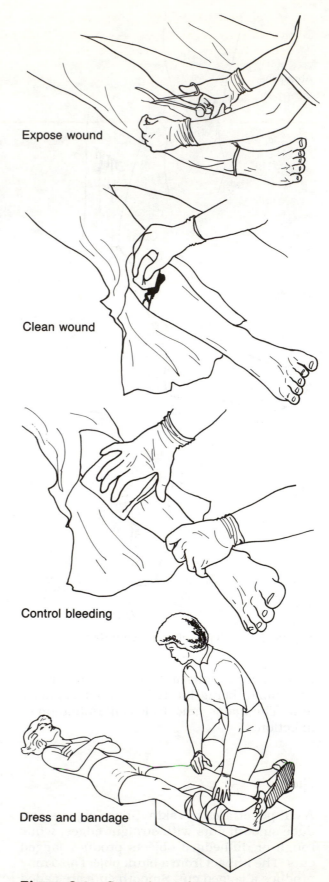

Expose wound

Clean wound

Control bleeding

Dress and bandage

Figure 6.4. General care for open wounds.

they have chemicals that may irritate exposed tissues. Commercial liquid soaps are available for general wound cleaning. If necessary you can use sterile saline solution or 3% hydrogen peroxide to cleanse wounds.

Dressing and Bandaging Wounds

Do not let an open wound go untreated. All open wounds should be cared for by applying a dressing and bandage. Dressings should be sterile. Bandages do not have to be sterile but should be very clean. Most commercially prepared gauze bandages are aseptic, that is, all foreign debris has been removed.

The following definitions apply to dressings and bandages (see Figure 6.5):

- *Dressing*. This is the material applied directly to a wound to help control bleeding and to prevent further contamination.
- *Bulky dressing*. These large dressings supply bulk to help control serious bleeding. You can make a bulky dressing by building up layers of small gauze dressings, or you can use commercial bulky dressings (universal, or multitrauma dressings). Although they are not sterile, individually wrapped sanitary napkins can be used as bulky dressings when open-wound bleeding is profuse. Avoid placing the adhesive surface against the skin and wound surface.
- *Occlusive dressing*. This commercially prepared, sterile plastic dressing is used for open chest and abdominal wounds

and for severed neck veins. It is used to help form an airtight seal.
- *Bandage*. This material is used to hold a dressing in place and to help immobilize the wound edges.
- *Self-adhesive bandage strip ("band-aid")*. This is a combination of dressing and bandage and is limited in use to minor, small wounds whose bleeding has been controlled. Elastic bandage strips are useful for covering minor cuts on the knuckles.

Dressing Wounds

Sterile dressings are available as individually wrapped sterile gauze pads. The most useful size is 4 square inches and is referred to as a "4 by 4." Many other sizes exist, including 2 by 4s and 4 by 8s. When removing a dressing from its wrapper, touch only the corner of the pad to ensure a sterile surface.

The following rules apply to the dressing of most wounds:

- *Use sterile materials*. If no sterile dressings are available, use the cleanest cloth material that is available at the scene (e.g., sheets or handkerchiefs).
- *Cover the entire wound surface*. Do not leave any of the wound exposed. It is best to cover the area immediately around the wound as well.
- *Control bleeding*. Do not bandage a dressing in place until bleeding has been controlled. (The exception is the pressure dressing described in chapter 5.) Use direct pressure over the top of the dressing to help control bleeding.
- *Leave dressings in place*. Do not remove dressings even if they are blood soaked as this may restart the bleeding or cause additional damage at the wound site. Instead, put new dressings over the top of the existing ones.

Bandaging

There is a variety of commercial bandages available, including self-adherent roller bandages, gauze bandages, and adhesive tape. When these materials are not available, cloth cravats can be used to tie the dressing in place. However, if you use a cravat, do not place the knot over the wound.

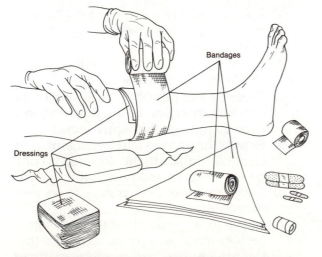

Figure 6.5. A variety of dressings and bandages are available.

Do not use elastic bandages that are meant for bruise, strain, and sprain care. These bandages too often prove to be constriction bands that interfere with or stop circulation.

The most useful bandage is the self-adherent, form-fitting, gauze roller bandage. Before this was invented, bandaging was a highly developed art form that required the right pattern and number of turns for different areas of the body. The roller bandage has all but eliminated the need to know specialized bandaging techniques for wound care.

The following rules apply to bandaging dressings in place:

- *Apply the bandage using the correct tension.* You must bandage snugly over the wound site, but the process should not restrict blood flow. The bandage is too tight if the athlete complains of numbness, tingling sensations, or pain associated with the bandage. Cold skin beyond the wound site and pale or blue coloring indicate that the bandaging is too tight. At the same time, make certain not to bandage too loosely. The dressing should not move around or slip off the wound but should be tight enough to keep the edges of the wound close together, thus promoting healing.
- *Tape any loose ends.* Bandage so that the gauze, cloth, or tape cannot get caught on objects when the athlete moves or is moved. Tape the end of a gauze wrap in place.
- *Leave the tips of fingers and toes exposed.* Changes in skin color at the fingertips and the tips of toes usually indicate a change in circulation. You must be able to assess circulation after bandaging is completed.
- *Leave some dressing exposed.* Avoid covering the dressing completely with tape. It is important for the wound to "breathe." In addition, do *not* wrap adhesive tape completely around a body part as this may cut off circulation.

Bandaging Joint Wounds

Wounds on major joints require special consideration. A small wound that has little bleeding can be treated by following the procedures for general wound care and by applying a bandaid (strip, circular, or rectangular). However, if wound care requires the use of gauze dressings and self-adherent roller bandages, several problems may occur. In your attempt to secure the dressing properly, take care to apply the bandage without binding the skin or cutting off circulation. Unless the bandage is secured properly, there is no guarantee that the dressing you applied will stay in place when the athlete moves.

If the wound is serious, make certain that the EMS system is being alerted and follow the general rules for wound care, dressing, and bandaging. Immobilize the limb so that the joint cannot be moved, treat for shock, and monitor the athlete until more highly trained help can take over.

WARNING:

A laceration across a joint surface requires special care if the wound edges move apart when the athlete bends and straightens the joint. The wound should be evaluated by a physician for possible suturing.

For joint wounds that are not serious, you can apply a figure-eight bandage to hold the dressing. This procedure works well for injuries to the elbows, wrists, knees, and ankles. Once bleeding is controlled and the wound properly dressed, you should use a self-adherent roller bandage to complete the figure eight (see Figure 6.6):

1. Make several turns around the limb so that the bandage overlaps the top edge of the dressing.
2. Cross the dressing diagonally.
3. Circle the limb below the joint.
4. Cross the dressing diagonally and in the opposite direction of the first diagonal (this completes the figure eight).
5. Repeat the process (circle, diagonal, circle, diagonal) until the dressing is completely covered and reasonably secure.
6. Tape the end of the bandage to prevent unwrapping.
7. Check to be certain that the bandage is neither too loose nor too tight and that the athlete can use the joint without

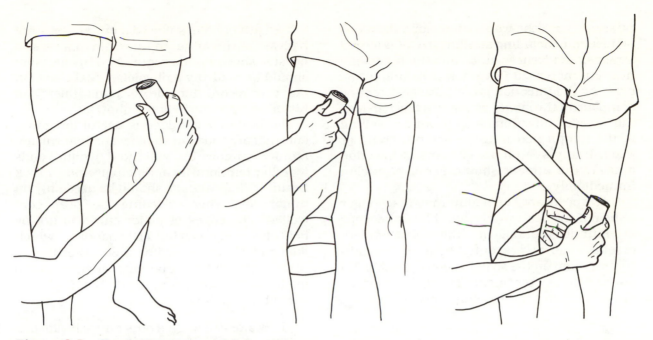

Figure 6.6. Bandaging across a joint.

causing the dressing to slip. Remember, there must be an adequate distal pulse in the affected limb.

Treating Specific Types of Wounds

As a coach you are likely to be faced with treating numerous open wounds. Suggestions for treating scratches and scrapes, cuts, puncture wounds, and avulsions are presented in the following pages.

Scratches and Scrapes

The principles of general wound care apply to treating most scratches. Some scrapes and combinations of scrapes and scratches may present special problems if the wound is dirty. It is not easy to clean this type of wound, particularly when debris is "ground in." This is a common problem for outdoor track-and-field events and for team sports played on natural surface.

Begin by warning the athlete that washing may hurt somewhat but that a thorough cleaning is necessary to prevent infection. Then gently scrub the wound with soap and water, using a sterile gauze pad to sweep away debris. Be careful, however, as pressure on the wound surface may be painful for the athlete. After

washing, rinse the area thoroughly with tepid water.

If a small wound remains dirty after washing, moisten a sterile pad with 3% hydrogen peroxide and clean the wound again. Tell the athlete what you are doing and why it is necessary. Alert him or her to possible "stings" and a little pain. The peroxide will foam and loosen dirt and will also act as a mild antiseptic. Do not apply peroxide if a large area of the skin is involved as this may be very painful for the athlete. In fact, the immediate care for all large wounds is to dress and bandage the wound and have a nurse or physician cleanse the wound.

WARNING:

Keep hydrogen peroxide away from the eyes.

If the athlete is a child, he or she may be more worried about showing a reaction to the pain of wound cleansing than about the wound itself. Provide the athlete with privacy and talk with him or her as you work.

Scratches and scrapes should form scabs and heal quickly; if they do not, insist that the athlete see a physician. During the healing process, check the wound daily for indications of infection, including swelling, redness (or red streaks), tenderness, and the athlete sensing heat (an increase in skin temperature) in the area. As the infection grows, the athlete may complain of throbbing pain and a feverish feeling. Serious infections may produce swelling of the lymph nodes in the armpit, groin, or neck. If any symptoms or signs of infection appear, the athlete should see a physician immediately.

A scrape located on a joint may take longer to heal if the scab cracks and bleeds because of continued motion. Once the scab is formed, cracking can be prevented by applying antiseptic cream on the scab to keep it flexible. Do not use greasy ointment. The site should be dressed during the healing process.

Cuts

General wound-care procedures apply to treating cuts. Your most important job is to control bleeding. The pressure dressing described in chapter 5 is an effective method for dealing with bleeding from a cut, or you may use direct pressure or direct pressure with elevation. Most bleeding can be controlled within 5 minutes.

If the wound is minor, it can be washed by applying mild soap and water with a sterile gauze pad. Wash the cut lengthwise to prevent additional damage to the wound at its edges, to keep debris from catching on the edge of the wound, and to prevent the restart of bleeding. Rinse thoroughly after washing.

Do not wash deep cuts or those with bleeding that is difficult to control. These injuries require a physician's attention. Any cut deeper than 1/8 inch or longer than 1/2 inch, a cut to the face, or a large cut on a joint is best treated by a physician. Serious cuts may require stitching, which must be done within 6 hours of the injury for normal healing to take place.

WARNING:

Do *not* open the cut to determine its depth or to see if it is clear. This may cause additional tissue damage or start serious bleeding. If you are in doubt about the severity or type of a cut, control bleeding, dress and bandage, and have the athlete see a physician.

If an athlete has suffered a cut and has not had an antitetanus shot within 5 years, a booster shot may be required. This decision should be made by a physician. Make certain that your records include when the athlete had his or her last antitetanus shot.

The butterfly bandage is useful for minor cuts that are wide but shallow and that will not require stitches. It will hold wound ends together temporarily and help promote quick healing. This bandage should be used only on minor cuts where bleeding has been controlled. The edges of major cuts will not be held effectively by a butterfly bandage, which does not control bleeding well. (Bleeding is best controlled by standard methods.) To make and to apply a butterfly bandage, you should do the following:

1. Make two angled cuts on each side of a small piece of adhesive tape, forming two triangles that are held together at their tips (see Figure 6.7). These are the "wings" of the butterfly.
2. Stick one wing on the side of the wound, then pinch the edges of the cut together. Do not overlap or roll the damaged tissues.
3. Pull the other wing tight and press it into place on the opposite side of the cut.
4. Apply a sterile gauze pad over the wound and secure it with a gauze roller bandage.

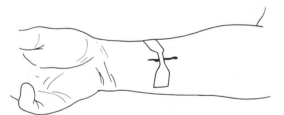

Figure 6.7. The butterfly bandage.

Puncture Wounds

The severity of a puncture wound is difficult to assess. It can be deep and cause serious tissue damage yet show little bleeding. The wound may appear to be free of the object causing the puncture, but a piece of that object may remain. The object causing the puncture sometimes appears to be embedded in the skin when it actually extends into the bone or has passed through the body part to produce an exit wound. Since skin and other soft tissues compress, the puncture may be deeper than the length of the object. For example, never assume that a spike wound goes no deeper than the length of the spike.

When assessing a puncture wound, you should consider the cause of injury (being spiked, minor fall onto the object, major fall, and so on), the object causing the puncture (sprinter's spike, jagged glass, splinter, and so on), the location of the wound, bleeding, and whether an object is impaled in the wound.

WARNING:

Do *not* squeeze a puncture wound to make it bleed. This may force contaminants deeper into the wound. Do not try to clean a deep puncture or use hydrogen peroxide to cleanse a puncture wound; rather, make certain that the EMS system is alerted, then control bleeding, dress, bandage, and treat for shock.

To care for minor puncture wounds without impaled objects, follow the general principles of wound care. If the wound appears deep or if the mechanism of injury indicates that it may be deep, do not wash the wound. Clear its surface, control bleeding, dress and bandage, and get the athlete to a physician. Any athlete needing an antitetanus shot or booster will have to see a physician after receiving a puncture wound.

Wounds containing impaled objects require special care. If an object such as a wood splinter or glass fragment is confined to the surface of the skin, it may be removed prior to dressing the wound. Forced removal of the object may sever surrounding tissue such as blood vessels, muscles, nerves, or ligaments. If the object is small and offers no resistance, it is probably safe to remove it. If you meet resistance, leave the object in place.

When a small impaled object is in the surface of the skin, it can be lifted out using sterilized tweezers. If it is just below the skin, it can be removed with the tip of a sterilized needle. To remove the object, you should take the following steps:

1. Clean the wound area with soap and water. Skip this step if part of the object is above the skin surface. You do not want to move the object or push it deeper into the skin.
2. Sterilize the instrument by soaking it in isopropyl alcohol or by heating it in a flame. Hold the heated instrument and let it cool before using.
3. Apply isopropyl alcohol to a sterile gauze pad and wipe the wound surface.
4. Remove the object.
5. Check to be sure that all foreign debris is removed.
6. Clean, dress, and bandage the wound.

Serious wounds with impaled objects are rare in sports, but they do occur. The athlete may fall on an object or have a piece of equipment or apparatus break and impale him or her with a sharp or jagged edge. The chances of an athlete being *impaled* by an object are greatly reduced when you properly manage the placement of sideline equipment and the condition of apparatus. Additional information about your legal responsibilities can be found in the ACEP Level 2 Sport Law Course described in the front of this book.

Do *not* remove an impaled object. To do so will likely cause additional injury and start major bleeding. Never pull an athlete off an impaled object, for the same dangers exist. The exception to this rule is when an object has punctured the cheek wall. Such an object may become loose in the oral cavity and become an airway obstruction.

Care for an athlete with an impaled object by placing padding around the impaled object to restrict its movement. Alert the EMS system of the injury and treat the athlete for shock.

Avulsions

Avulsions are rare in sports, but they do occur. If the skin is torn loose but is not completely severed, take these steps:

1. Make certain that the needed health care professional is alerted. If there is serious bleeding, a large section of tissue is avulsed, or the avulsion is facial skin, have the EMS system alerted.
2. Do *not* try to clean this type of wound but simply clear the surface.
3. *Gently* fold the skin back to its normal position.
4. Control bleeding, dress, and bandage. You may have to use bulky dressings and a gauze pressure bandage.

When the skin, the tip of the nose, a part of the external ear, or a small part of the fingertip or tip of the toe is cut or torn completely from the body, do the following:

1. Make certain that the EMS system is alerted.
2. Control bleeding by using a bulky pressure dressing.
3. Reassure the athlete and treat for shock.
4. Save the avulsed part in a plastic bag or plastic wrap. Label the bag and keep the part as cool as possible. Do *not* allow it to freeze or come into contact with ice or water.

Changing Dressings

The first person to provide care usually dresses and bandages a wound and does not need to be concerned about when to change the dressing. As a coach, you will probably have to do both the initial and the follow-up care. You should change a dressing at least once each day and when any of the following conditions exist:

- *The dressing is dirty.* This is most often the case when the athlete is allowed to return to the game.
- *The dressing is wet or has been wet.* This is bound to happen on the field or in the showers, but it can happen almost anywhere. It is difficult to keep most dressed wounds completely dry.
- *Bleeding has stopped.* Sometimes it is necessary to replace dried, blood-soaked dressings. This should be done only when bleeding has fully stopped and not while it is only being controlled.
- *Looking for infection.* The early signs of infection can be missed unless you look at the wound. After inspection, the wound needs a new dressing.
- *Tape has been used.* Some types of band-aid and adhesive tape do not allow air to pass through and reach the skin. The skin will turn white and become soft and moist.
- *Dressings or bandages fail.* Not every dressing or bandage will stay in place, particularly when the athlete returns to action.

The major problem with changing a dressing is when the scab sticks to the gauze. If the dressing is pulled away roughly, the scab may break and bleeding may restart. If a scab sticks to the dressing, wet a piece of gauze with 3% hydrogen peroxide, place it on top of the dressing, and let it soak for a minute or two. The peroxide should soften the scab, allowing you to remove the dressing. Do not apply the peroxide near the eyes. Also, do not use warm water in place of peroxide as this may cause the tissue to become soft and moist and thus delay healing.

Returning to Action

If the athlete has suffered a serious open wound, a physician should decide when he or she can return to participate in practice and events. In the case of minor wounds, you will probably be making that decision. The athlete should be rested if he or she is experiencing pain, if the injury significantly limits performance, or if activity could reopen the healing wound. Rest is appropriate when the discomfort of the injury is taking away the athlete's enjoyment of the activity.

Injuries to the face should be allowed to heal completely before the athlete is exposed to the possibility of reinjury. Scarring of facial injuries is greatly reduced if the wound is not reopened.

SUMMARY AND RECOMMENDATIONS

Damage to soft tissues can be classified as closed wounds and open wounds. Remember these key points of providing wound care:

1. Most closed wounds are bruises, but you must stay alert for signs of internal injury and bleeding. Moderate and severe bruises can be treated with the RICE method. Most mild bruises require no special treatment; however, the application of ice is helpful.
2. If the bruised athlete has moderate to severe pain, point tenderness, stiffness or loss of function, or lasting muscle spasms, you should immobilize the injured part and be sure the athlete is cared for by a physician.

3. Most open wounds can be cared for by exposing the wound, clearing or cleaning the wound surface, controlling bleeding, applying a dressing that covers the entire wound, and securing the dressing with a bandage.

4. Remember to keep the injured athlete lying still. An injured limb can be elevated if there are no indications of fracture.

5. Do not remove a dressing once it is in place on the wound or over other blood-soaked dressings.

6. If you are in doubt about the seriousness (determined by size and depth) or cleanliness of an open wound, seek medical assistance. Any wound with bleeding that is difficult to control requires a physician's attention.

7. All wounds with impaled objects or avulsions must be cared for by a physician.

8. Stay on the alert for the symptoms and signs of infection and change dressings frequently to observe the wound site. Allow an athlete to return to action only when activity is pain free and will not reopen the wound.

Chapter 7
Soft-Tissue Injuries—The Head and Neck

This chapter continues the discussion of soft-tissue injuries. There are many potential problems associated with head and neck injuries, including skull fractures, brain injury, spinal column fractures and dislocations, and spinal cord damage. For now, the discussion will be limited to the soft tissues; however, you must be on the alert for more serious injuries. Chapter 12 will discuss skull, brain, and spinal injuries.

THE SCALP AND FACE

Whenever an injury, no matter how minor, occurs to the head, make certain that the athlete has an open airway. Because there are so many blood vessels located close to the skin of the scalp and face, it is easy to concentrate on bleeding and miss the early signs of partial airway obstruction. Likewise, being over-concerned with bleeding may cause you to miss signs that indicate serious injury to the bones of the skull or the neck. Remember to consider the mechanism of injury. For example, a tennis ball hitting the cheek will probably cause a bruise, while a baseball may fracture the cheekbone.

This does not mean that bleeding should be thought of as a minor problem. It will have to be controlled, but keep your mind open to other possible injuries. You can begin to control bleeding while making your assessment of the injury. Avoid direct pressure over the injury site until you have ruled out the possibility of fractures and other serious injuries.

Bleeding from the scalp and face can be profuse even when the injury is minor. Do not use bleeding as the only sign of serious injury. Again, the mechanism of injury and other signs will have to be considered.

Most injuries to the scalp and face should receive the same care as that for the typical soft-tissue injury. There are five major exceptions:

- Do not apply compression to ice packs or cold packs being used to treat simple bruises.
- Do not clear the surface of a scalp wound if the mechanism of injury or other signs indicate that there may be damage to the skull bones. Do not attempt to pull debris from the wound as this may restart bleeding. A minor scratch may be cleaned, but more serious open wounds should *never* be washed by the coach but by a physician. If the wound is deeper than you suspect and the underlying bone has been fractured, washing could lead to a serious brain infection.
- Do not apply finger or hand pressure to a head wound if there are indications of a possible skull fracture.
- Do *not* apply direct pressure to a cut or a punctured eyeball.
- Do not use pressure or packing to stop the flow of clear or bloody fluids from the nose or ears.

Care of Scalp Wounds

Simple bruises to the scalp can be cared for with ice packs or cold packs without compression. Although this method is not very effective because of the number of surface blood vessels, it does provide some comfort. Continue to observe the athlete for changes in his or her state of awareness and for any changes at the injury site. Do not dismiss a "goose egg" by considering this a minor sign. Be sure to check for more serious injuries. Also, check periodically for clear or bloody fluids in the nose and ears that may be the release of cerebrospinal fluids, a major indication of skull fracture.

All deep, open scalp wounds and those associated with serious impacts should be treated by a physician. The basic steps for scalp-wound care include the following:

1. Do not clear or clean the surface unless you are certain that the wound is a minor scratch.
2. Control bleeding by holding a dressing over the wound. If there are any signs of skull fracture, do *not* apply pressure over the wound site. The loose dressing will help promote the reduction of blood flow.
3. After controlling the bleeding, wrap a self-adherent roller bandage around the head to secure the dressing as shown in Figure 7.1. If there are any indications of more serious head injury or of neck and spinal injury, simply control the bleeding, stabilize the head (see p. 137), and wait for more highly trained help to arrive.
4. If there are no serious injuries, position the athlete with the head and shoulders elevated.

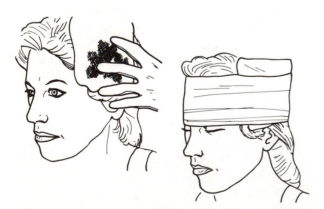

Figure 7.1. Treating scalp wounds.

A triangular bandage can be used to secure dressings placed over scalp wounds. This is a useful method when the wound is to the top of the head (see Figure 7.2).

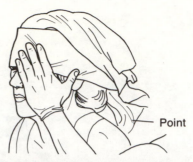

1. Create a 2-inch hem along the base of the triangular cloth by folding the material. Keep the folded edge out as you position the bandage on the athlete's forehead. The point of the bandage should hang down behind the rear of the athlete's head.

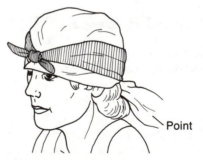

2. Pull the ends of the bandage behind the athlete's head. Tie these ends together over top of the point of the bandage.

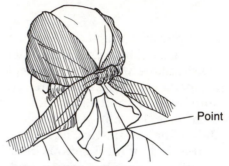

3. Draw the ends to the front of the athlete's head. Tie these ends together, avoiding undue pressure on the athlete's forehead.

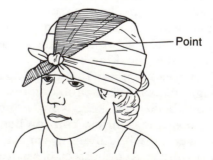

4. Bring the rear point of the bandage forward over the top of the athlete's head. Tuck this point under the tied ends.

Figure 7.2. The triangular bandage.

Care of Facial Wounds

Simple bruises on the face can be cared for with ice or cold packs. Do not apply compression. Keep checking the athlete for an open airway, altered states of awareness, and signs of fractures. Look several times for clear or bloody fluids in the nose and ears and have all deep or long, open wounds treated by a physician. You should alert the EMS system for all injuries that involve impaled objects.

The basic care for open facial injuries includes the following:

1. Check for breathing problems, neck and spinal injury, and more serious head wounds.
2. Control bleeding with direct pressure. Avoid pressure over possible fractures.
3. Dress and bandage the wound. Do not block the airway.

CARE OF EYE INJURIES

The eye is a delicate organ on which we tend to rely heavily. In fact, sight is perhaps our most dominating sense. Figure 7.3 illustrates the structures of the eye. It is important that you be aware of these structures and can distinguish between them.

Some eye-injury care may be complicated by the presence of contact lenses; however, most initial care is effective when they are left in place. You should not attempt to remove contact lenses unless you have been specifically trained to do so. There are four types of lenses: hard, flexible (soft), extended wear, and scleral. (You can obtain additional information on vision and contact lenses from the American Optometric Association, 243 North Lindbergh Boulevard, St. Louis, MO 63141.)

Common injuries to the eye include bruises ("black eyes"), foreign objects in the eye, and cuts and scratches to the lid or globe. Some of these injuries will require dressing and bandaging. When it is necessary to bandage an eye, you will need to bandage both eyes to reduce eye movement. If you leave the uninjured eye uncovered, it will move to follow the objects it sees. The injured eye will move with the uninjured one in *sympathetic movement*, that is, duplicating the movements of the uncovered eye, and this may aggravate the injury.

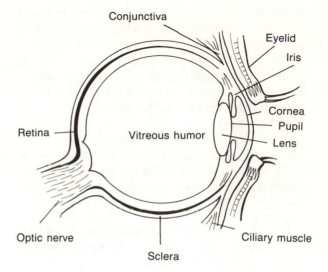

Figure 7.3. The eye.

Bruises

The mechanism of injury and the force of the blow are the key factors in determining the care for a bruised eye. If there is a possibility of more serious injuries, treat the injury as if the athlete has head and neck injuries and wait for an EMS response. Do *not* allow movement of the head. Alert the EMS system for quick transport if

- the iris, or the colored area around the pupil, is not clearly visible; or
- there is blood between the clear structure over the top of the iris, the cornea, and the iris.

Simple bruises on the globe, lid, and in regions around the eye can be cared for by applying an ice pack or a cold pack without compression. Be sure to place a dry cloth or a few sterile gauze pads between the pack and the eye. The pack should be applied for 30 minutes, and the athlete should be allowed to remove it periodically for the sake of comfort. If vision is limited by swelling, the athlete should rest for at least 24 hours. If the athlete complains of distorted vision, he or she should consult a physician as soon as possible.

Foreign Objects

In most cases, the athlete's tears will wash away foreign debris in the eye. Encourage the athlete to remain at rest with both eyes closed and not to rub them. Do *not* wash an athlete's eyes if there are cuts or puncture wounds to the eyeball. Do not probe into the eye socket, and *never* attempt to remove an object on the cornea. Cover both eyes and have the athlete seen by a physician without delay. Arrange for EMS transport.

When safe to do so, objects can be washed from the eyes using clean, tepid water or sterile saline solution. To wash the eye, you should follow these procedures (see Figure 7.4):

1. Position the athlete so that water can be poured from the nasal corner of the eye and washed across the entire globe.
2. Hold the upper lash with your thumb and forefinger.
3. Fold the upper lid over an applicator stick.
4. Have the athlete look down to expose the upper surface of the eye and to resist watching your activities.
5. Apply water to the nasal corner. Several cups of water will wash most debris from the eye. While washing, direct the athlete to look from side to side and up and down.

If debris remains in the eye, dress and bandage both eyes and have the athlete consult a physician.

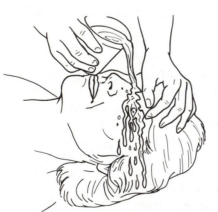

Figure 7.4. Washing debris from the eye.

Cuts and Scratches

Minor scratches to the eyelid require that bleeding be controlled with a gauze dressing. Scratches to the eyeball are seldom serious unless they involve the cornea. In these cases,

the athlete should be treated by a physician or qualified eye specialist.

Take great care when treating an athlete with a cut eyeball. It is very difficult to tell the depth of the wound. Arrange for EMS transport. *Never* apply direct pressure to a cut eyeball. There is a jellylike fluid called the *vitreous humor* that fills the back chamber of the eye, and pressure may force this fluid out through the cut. The vitreous humor cannot be replaced either naturally or artificially. Its loss could mean blindness. Place loose dressings over the eye to help control bleeding. Do the same for puncture wounds that do not have impaled objects.

There are some less common eye injuries that may require your care, including burns, impaled objects, and avulsions of the eyelid and eyeball.

Burns

Light burns ("snow blindness") occur from exposure to reflected sunlight and are seen in outdoor winter sports and water sports. Instruct the athlete to close his or her eyes and place dark patches over the eyelids. You can use several layers of gauze pads covered by dark plastic. A gauze roller bandage can be used to hold these patches in place. The athlete may experience extreme pain that is usually delayed 3-5 hours after the first complaint. Arrange for the athlete to be seen by a physician as soon as possible.

Chemical burns, other than the minor irritation caused by swimming pool chemicals, are seldom seen in sports activities, especially since lime is no longer used to line fields. If a chemical gets into the athlete's eye, wash both eyes with water. Current recommendations call for a 20-minute flowing wash for acids and for alkali (lime). (These recommendations have recently been updated in response to the inability of the observer to detect the chemical nature and contamination level of the materials involved. Play it safe.) If pain returns, continue washing, then have the athlete close his or her eyes. Apply loose, dry dressings over the eyelids. All athletes with chemical burns to the eyes should be transported by the EMS system to a physician.

Impaled Objects

It is possible for someone to fall on some hidden wooden debris on a playing field or be struck in the eye when a stick or a bat breaks. These accidents may lead to an object becoming impaled in the eye. *Never* exert pressure on an impaled object but have the EMS system alerted and stabilize the object. This can be done by placing a 3-inch roll of gauze on each side of the object (see Figure 7.5).

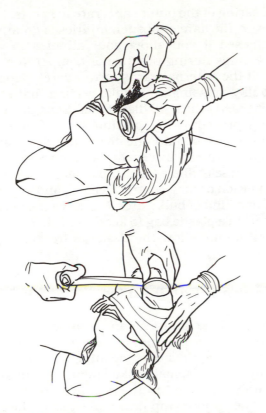

Figure 7.5. Care for an object impaled in the eye.

Make a shield for the eye by placing a slightly crushed drinking cup or paper cone on top of the dressings. Do not let this shield come in contact with the impaled object. Use a self-adherent roller bandage to hold the shield and dressings in place. Cover the uninjured eye with dressing pads secured with roller dressing. Throughout the entire process, continually reassure the athlete, as eye injuries require a great deal of emotional support.

Avulsions

An eye that is pulled fully or partially from its socket is called an *avulsed eye*. In some cases, only the cornea is avulsed. An avulsed eye may be caused by the eye being hit in a towel-snapping melee. Such an event would certainly turn fun into a near tragedy. We recommend

that you warn your athletes of the dangers of this type of horseplay and deal with its occurrence harshly.

If you need to care for an eye avulsion, do *not* attempt to replace the eye. Care is basically the same as that for an impaled object in the eye. It is easier to bandage the injury if the stabilizing gauze rolls are replaced with a "doughnut ring," which is made from a 2-inch roll of self-adherent roller bandage. Wrap the gauze around three of your fingers and your thumb. Make seven or eight turns, spreading your fingers to adjust the size of the opening. It must be large enough to fit around the avulsed eye without touching it. Remove the doughnut from your fingers and wrap the rest of the roll through the hole, around the side of the bandage, and back through the hold. Continue this process until you have finished the roll or have obtained the correct thickness (see Figure 7.6).

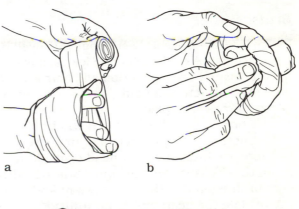

a   b

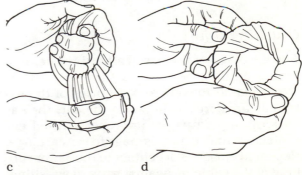

c   d

Figure 7.6. A doughnut ring can be used for eye care.

Partially torn eyelids should be cared for with loose dressings. If the lid is fully avulsed, remember to save the part. Cover both eyes with dressings and secure them with a roller bandage.

EAR INJURIES

Injuries can occur to the external and the internal ear. An external injury may or may not be associated with more severe head and neck injuries, but internal injuries usually are. Regardless of the type of injury, if the athlete complains of distorted or diminished hearing or of a total loss of hearing in one or both ears, alert the EMS system for immediate transport.

External Ear Injuries

External ear injuries include bruises, crushing injuries to the cartilage of the ear, scratches, cuts, and avulsions. In most cases, all that is needed is basic care provided by the coach. Usually, if any problem does not respond well to such care immediately, a physician will have to see the athlete.

Bruises

There is very little soft tissue that can swell in a bruised ear. A cold pack or an ice pack is still useful because its application will help relieve pain. The athlete can hold it in place by hand and remove and replace the pack for comfort. This is probably all the care that will be necessary unless the mechanism of injury is severe or there are indications of head or neck injury. In these cases alert the appropriate health care professional or the EMS system and treat the athlete for head and neck injury.

Crushing Injury

The cartilage of the ear is a hard tissue. It is discussed here because cartilage damage is often related to soft-tissue injuries of the external ear. Forceful blows to the ear, the ear striking apparatus, or improperly fitted ear protectors may cause damage to ear cartilage. Repeated episodes of contact to the ear or rubbing of the ear (e.g., against mats in wrestling) may damage the cartilage and produce *cauliflower ear*.

Never consider damage to cartilage to be minor. The athlete will have to see a physician. Your care procedures should include applying a bulky dressing over the top of the injured ear.

Scratches and Cuts

Clean the wound and apply a dressing and bandage. If the ear is torn, treat the injury as you would an avulsion.

Avulsions

Tearing of the outer ear is rare in sports. However, the danger of such injuries is greatly increased if you allow your athletes to wear earrings during practice or competition.

If the external ear is torn severely, apply a bulky dressing and make certain that someone alerts the EMS dispatcher. Start the dressing procedure by placing several layers of dressings behind the torn ear. Next, apply bulky dressings over the ear and secure them with a self-adherent roller bandage. When a full avulsion occurs, control bleeding and apply the same kind of bulky dressing. Save the avulsed part in a plastic bag to keep it dry. Keep it cool, but do not allow the tissue to freeze.

Internal Ear Injuries

Internal ear injuries can be minor or severe. Pain may or may not be present. Any pain in the ear requires that the athlete be seen by a physician. If spinal or skull injuries occur at the same time, tend to those injuries first.

The major symptoms and signs of the injury determine the care. These include "clogged" ear, bleeding from the ear, and fluids draining from the ear.

Ear Pain and Hearing Impairment

A complaint of hearing impairment or "clogged ear" could signal potential problems. For example, if the complaint occurs following trauma to the head, check for drainage of clear or bloody fluid from the ear canal or nose. If these fluids are present, alert the EMS system, keep the athlete at rest, and treat for a possible head injury. The athlete should not be allowed to shake the head for any reason.

Intense pain followed by hearing loss and possibly severe dizzying and nausea may indicate rupture of the eardrum. The athlete should be evaluated by a physician and, if a swimmer or diver, should not be allowed in the pool until medically cleared.

Additional causes of ear pain and hearing impairment include the following, each of which requires care by a medical professional.

- Middle ear inflammation
- Upper respiratory infection
- Seasonal allergy
- Swimmer's ear
- Earwax build-up

WARNING:

Never probe into the ear. Seek medical attention for athletes suffering from ear pain or hearing impairment.

Bleeding

Bleeding from the ear does not always indicate a serious problem. In sport activities, it usually means a scratch to the external ear canal. If there is a flow of blood or if your visual inspection shows blood in the canal, arrange for EMS transport. Do *not* attempt to pack the canal with cotton as this could cause serious internal damage or infection. Instead, dress and bandage the external ear. Any bleeding from the ear related to head injury or not associated with a minor scratch requires you to alert the EMS system.

Draining Fluids

Clear or bloody fluids in the ear or draining from the ear mean that there could be a skull fracture. Alert the EMS system, treat for head injury, and apply a loose dressing to the external ear. Do *not* pack the ear with cotton. If the flow is cerebrospinal fluid, attempting to stop the flow with packs could lead to a serious infection.

NOSE INJURIES

There are three major concerns with nasal injuries. You must be certain that (a) there is an open airway, (b) there are no serious head or spinal injuries, and (c) bleeding is controlled.

External scratches, scrapes, and cuts are treated using the general care methods for soft-tissue injuries. Special consideration must be given to nosebleeds, fluids draining from the nose, and avulsions.

Nosebleeds

Nosebleeds are common sport injuries and can occur because of contact in wrestling, basketball, football, and in virtually every sport. The amount of bleeding from the nose can range from minor to profuse. Unless the mechanism of injury indicates a serious facial injury, nasal bleeding is usually easy to control. Do *not* pack the nostrils, but let the athlete sit and lean forward to keep blood from draining down the airway. Next, have the athlete pinch his or her nostrils shut. This will control most bleeding. The previously accepted technique of tilting back the athlete's head is contraindicated as this could easily lead to the aspiration of blood and the athlete choking. The appropriate technique is illustrated in Figure 7.7.

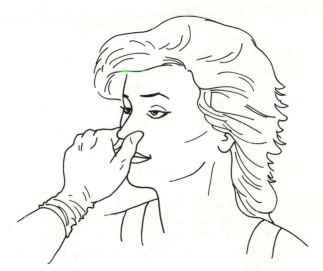

Figure 7.7. Care for a simple nosebleed.

In some cases, control of a nosebleed can be improved by placing some rolled gauze between the upper lip and gum and having the athlete press against the bandage with his or her fingers or stretch the lip tightly against the bandage. An ice pack or a cold pack applied to the nose may help to stop the flow.

If bleeding is profuse or long lasting or if the athlete has a history of nosebleeds, a physician's care is needed. Keep the nostrils pinched shut while awaiting transport.

Draining Fluids

Clear or bloody fluids draining from an injured nose indicate a possible skull fracture. Alert the EMS system and treat for head injury. Never assume that the clear flow is from the sinuses even if the athlete has a history of sinus problems. Do *not* pack the nose. You may, however, apply a loose dressing.

MOUTH INJURIES

Your main duty in providing care for mouth injuries is to ensure an open airway, which usually involves little more than positioning the athlete for proper drainage. When the athlete is free of other injuries, he or she can be seated with the head tilted forward to provide drainage. If the athlete is lying down, your actions depend on the severity of his or her other injuries. If there are no indications of neck, spinal, or severe head injuries but you are concerned about injury to the extremities or trunk, keep the athlete at rest and turn his or her head to the side for drainage.

The most common soft-tissue injuries to the mouth include cuts to the lips, gums, tongue, and inner cheek. You may also see avulsed lips, perforated inner cheeks, and avulsed tongues.

Cut Lips and Gums

The lips and gums can be cut by contact with an external implement or by the athlete's own teeth being forced into the tissue. To care for these injuries, place a folded dressing between the lip and gum and position the athlete for drainage. It is best to allow 3-4 inches of dressing material to hang outside of the mouth to allow for quick removal should the athlete suffer a loss of consciousness. Monitor the athlete to be sure that the dressing is not swallowed. Minor bleeding can also be controlled by applying ice wrapped in sterile gauze. If bleeding is profuse or if there are signs of more serious injury, alert the EMS system.

Cut or Avulsed Tongue

These injuries, too, can be caused by external implements or the athlete's teeth. Those athletes who play their sport while sticking their tongue out between their teeth are particularly susceptible to these injuries.

Unless a cut to the tongue is very small, the athlete will have to see a physician. If bleeding continues or is profuse, the EMS system should be alerted, regardless of the size of the injury. Do *not* pack the mouth to control bleeding, but position the athlete for drainage. If an avulsion has occurred, you may find tissue in the mouth. Remove any fully avulsed tissue and save it as you would any avulsed tissue.

Cut and Perforated Inner Cheeks

Wounds to the inner cheek other than minor cuts will have to be cared for by a physician. If bleeding is profuse or cannot be controlled, alert the EMS system. To control bleeding, place rolled dressing between the wound and the athlete's teeth and position the athlete for drainage. Remember to allow 3-4 inches of dressing material to hang outside of the mouth in case you need to remove the dressing quickly.

INJURIES INVOLVING THE TEETH

Injuries of the teeth will be covered in this chapter because they are associated with injury to the soft tissues of the mouth. The most common injuries to the teeth include cracks and chips to the teeth and fillings and loose teeth and fillings. These injuries are often ignored unless the front teeth are involved, but this is a serious mistake. First, if the blow that caused the injury was strong enough to damage a tooth, it may have caused other damage. Be sure to check for head and neck injuries. Second, a dentist will want to examine the damage and will probably call for an X ray.

If the crack is deeper than you believe it to be or if the chip has caused damage deep in the tooth, an abscess may occur, causing the loss of the tooth. Professional care is needed for any injury involving the teeth.

Never assume that a loose tooth is a temporary problem that will correct itself. Professional care is needed to prevent loss of the tooth or abscess.

It is possible that a cracked tooth is ready to break off. If this happens while the athlete is involved in activity, the broken piece could be swallowed and obstruct the airway. For this reason, you should not let an athlete participate in activities if he or she has a cracked or loose tooth or filling. The athlete should see a dentist or oral surgeon as soon as possible.

Always check for dislodged teeth, crowns, bridges, and fillings when you inspect the mouth for injury. They must be removed to prevent possible airway obstruction.

It is a good policy (especially in contact sports) to have the athlete's dentist approve of participation if the athlete will practice or play while wearing dental appliances (crowns, bridges, dentures, or braces). Never let an athlete participate in activities if he or she is wearing a unilateral partial known as a Nesbit (some people call this a "spider"). A Nesbit (see Figure 7.8) is a one- or two-tooth partial that is held in place at four points. There have been cases of people swallowing Nesbits.

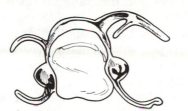

Figure 7.8. The Nesbit, or "spider" partial.

When a tooth is knocked out of its socket, it is called an avulsed tooth. If the avulsed tooth is still in the mouth, remove it immediately to avoid possible airway obstruction. Control bleeding from the socket by having the athlete bite down on a piece of gauze dressing placed over the socket. Leave 3-4 inches of the gauze outside of the athlete's mouth in case quick removal of the dressing is necessary. Do *not* stuff cotton packets in the socket as this can damage tissues and reduce the chances of the tooth being replanted successfully. It is impossible to have an unconscious person bite down, but if the athlete is unconscious and bleeding from the socket is profuse, gauze can be placed in the socket after immobilizing the head and neck (see chapter 12).

An avulsed tooth can be replanted. Save the dislodged tooth and have it transported with the athlete. It is critical that you *not* clean the tooth as this will most likely destroy microscopic structures needed for successful replanting. Keep the tooth wrapped in a moist dressing or in a small container of milk. The

athlete will have to see a dentist or oral surgeon as soon as possible. Most successful tooth replants take place within 30 minutes of the injury.

SOFT-TISSUE INJURIES OF THE NECK

The anatomy of the neck (see Figure 7.9) makes this body part susceptible to severe injury. Since the head is large and heavy (proportionally more so in children than in adults), injury to the head often involves the neck and vice versa. Injuries to the neck can involve spinal injuries, large-blood-vessel injuries, and airway obstruction. It is safest to assume that all neck injuries are very serious until you can prove otherwise. If you cannot tell how serious the injury is, assume that it is very serious and arrange for an EMS response. *All* injuries to the neck require you to assess the athlete for other injuries.

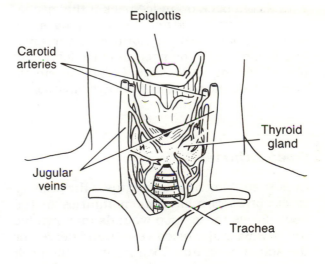

Figure 7.9. Anatomy of the neck.

Closed Injuries

When an athlete suffers a blunt injury to the neck (e.g., when hit by a ball, bat, arm, or leg), make certain that the airway is open and, if necessary, do a spinal assessment. Check carefully for injury to the larynx and trachea, which should be in their normal alignment. If anything seems wrong, alert the EMS system and treat for spinal and head injuries.

The symptoms and signs of a serious blunt injury to the neck include the following:

- Loss of voice or distorted voice
- Trachea deviated to the side
- Any sign of airway obstruction
- Bruises
- Depressions
- Swelling
- Pain
- Tenderness
- Muscle spasm
- Crackling sensations under the skin (These sensations come from air leaking out of the airway and becoming trapped in the soft tissues of the neck. The athlete may tell you that he or she feels this sensation or you might detect it with your fingertips while examining the injury site.)

The severity of a neck injury is not always immediately apparent. As tissues swell, airway obstruction may take place, so it is best to rest and monitor any athlete who has a blunt injury to the neck.

Simple bruises on the neck can be treated with a cold pack or an ice pack if the mechanism of injury is mild and the airway and spine appear undamaged. Do not use compression and do not leave the pack in place for a long period of time. Direct the athlete to remove and replace the pack, and always have someone monitor the athlete.

Open Injuries

Broken equipment or apparatus is the primary cause of sport-related open injuries to the neck. Since these open wounds may involve the airway, major blood vessels and nerves, or the spinal cord, any open injury of the neck other than minor scrapes, scratches, and cuts requires an EMS response. If the airway is damaged, be prepared to provide basic life support. Fortunately, open wounds to these structures are extremely rare. If you are faced with bleeding from a major neck artery or vein,

have someone call for an EMS response immediately while you attempt to control the bleeding with direct pressure applied to a bulky dressing. Hold the dressing firmly in place over the wound site without obstructing breathing. Do *not* apply pressure to both sides of the neck simultaneously.

SUMMARY AND RECOMMENDATIONS

When providing care for soft-tissue injuries to the head and neck, you must follow the general rules for wound care and remember the major exceptions to the rules:

1. When providing care for face wounds, always ensure an open airway. If there are no injuries to the skull, spine, or neck, position the athlete for drainage. Dress and bandage all open wounds.
2. You must take special care with eye wounds. Do *not* apply direct pressure to an open wound of the eye, wash the eye if there are open wounds, or remove impaled objects.
3. If you are caring for an ear wound, do *not* pack the ear canal to stop bleeding or the flow of fluids. Do *not* probe the ear.
4. Nose injuries require you to ensure an open airway. Control bleeding by positioning the athlete for drainage and pinching the nostrils shut. *Always* check for clear or bloody fluids in the nose and ears.
5. When caring for mouth injuries, be certain that there is an open airway and, when possible, adequate drainage. Remove any parts from broken or avulsed teeth to protect the airway.
6. Neck injuries can be very serious. When the neck is injured, you must assess the severity of the injury and look for other injuries, including those to the airway, major blood vessels, and spine.

Chapter 8
Soft-Tissue Injuries—The Trunk

The trunk consists of the chest, back, abdomen, and pelvis, with the shoulders and pelvic bones considered to be parts of the extremities. Because the trunk houses numerous vital organs and structures (see Figure 8.1), any injury to this area is potentially serious.

Possible soft-tissue injuries include those to the skin, muscles, blood vessels, nerves, fibrous membranes, internal organs and glands, breasts, and genitalia (external reproductive organs). Any severe injury to the trunk may also involve structures in the head, neck, and back.

CHEST INJURIES

Sport-related injuries to the chest rarely involve more than the soft tissues, and, when they do occur, the injuries are generally minor ones. Because the heart and lungs are in the

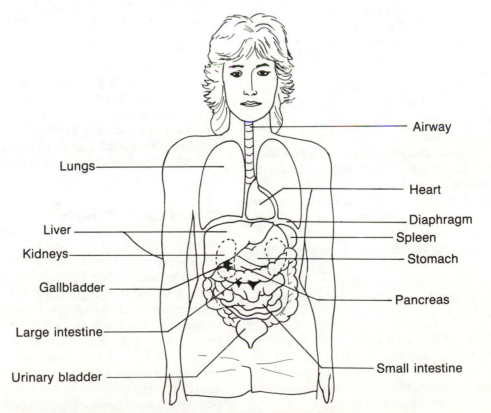

Figure 8.1. Many vital organs and structures in the trunk are subject to injury.

chest cavity and forces applied to the chest can affect the neck and spine, it is important that injuries to this region be assessed with the understanding that certain symptoms and signs indicate a possible emergency requiring immediate attention.

The detection of, and the proper care for, minor chest injuries is very important. Soft-tissue injuries can take the fun out of participation by causing pain and sometimes altering breathing patterns. If an athlete is allowed to play while having sore areas on the chest (including the flanks), he or she may attempt to protect these injured areas with the arms. The athlete is usually unaware of any change in body positioning or mechanics that serves to guard an injured area. This protective behavior can lead to additional injuries.

Symptoms and Signs of Chest Injury

Any injury to the chest, even if it appears to involve only soft tissues, must be considered to be serious if you detect any of the following:

- Changes in level of consciousness
- Difficult or painful breathing
- Coughing up of bright red frothy blood
- Any symptoms and signs of shock, especially a rapid weak pulse and skin-color changes
- Bulging (distended) neck veins
- Windpipe appearing pushed away from the injured side of the chest
- Any penetrating wound of the chest
- Any large bruise or area of bruises or a bruise associated with severe impact, compression, or a fall
- Unequal chest movements or the failure of the chest to expand and contract normally
- Pain on compression of the sides of the chest
- Crackling sensations under the skin reported by the athlete or felt during assessment

Any of these symptoms and signs requires immediate care, constant monitoring, and an EMS response as soon as possible. Be prepared for vomiting, changes in level of consciousness, and respiratory or cardiac arrest.

Open Chest Injuries

Simple cuts and scrapes to the skin of the chest can be cared for as described in chapter 6. The exception is any open wound that involves the nipples. In these cases, basic wound care should be provided and the athlete (male or female) attended to by a physician.

Open chest wounds are usually the result of the athlete falling or being throw onto a sharp object. On rare occasions, the breaking of equipment or apparatus may be the cause. Prevention—through proper maintenance of playing fields and surfaces and regular safety inspections of equipment—makes this type of injury a rare event.

The term "open chest wound" usually refers to an injury that has penetrated the chest wall. Any penetrating chest wound requires immediate on-the-scene physician or EMS intervention and transport to a medical facility due to the difficulty in assessing the depth of this type of wound. Never attempt to open a chest wound to determine its depth but assume that it is deep and call for the proper response. You should assess the athlete's vital signs, treat for shock, and monitor the athlete's condition until help arrives.

The dangers associated with penetrating chest wounds include the following:

- Direct injury to the heart, lungs, and great blood vessels
- Indirect injury to the heart, lungs, and great blood vessels caused by pressure changes and blood in the chest cavity
- Severe breathing problems (e.g., labored breathing and gasping) caused by pressure changes in the chest cavity

Closed Chest Injuries

A simple bruise to the chest can be cared for as described in chapter 6. If the mechanism of injury is such that you believe additional injuries may exist, symptoms and signs indicate other injuries, or the athlete's condition begins to worsen, an immediate EMS response and evaluation by a physician are necessary.

Most other types of closed chest injury are very severe and require you to maintain an open airway, provide basic cardiac life support when appropriate, have the EMS system alerted, treat for shock, and monitor the injured athlete.

If you suspect rib fractures, be on the alert for tension pneumothorax, which can occur if a lung is punctured. This condition occurs when air escapes from the lung and is trapped in the chest cavity. The excess pressure that is formed can collapse the lung and may damage the heart. Since the pressure cannot be released, respiratory arrest is a possibility.

Injuries caused by compression of the chest cavity, as seen in instances of "piling on" in football or rugby, body checking in ice hockey, or illegal body slams in wrestling, may produce serious injury to the lungs and/or heart. If your assessment reveals any of the symptoms or signs listed earlier for severe chest injury, take immediate action and make certain that the EMS dispatcher is alerted to the nature of the injury. While you await the arrival of medical assistance, maintain an open airway and treat the athlete for shock.

Injuries to the Breasts

Most injuries to the breast can be prevented by the female athlete wearing a properly fitted brassiere designed for athlete activities. Such a bra will help prevent injury associated with the vertical and lateral movements produced during running and jumping. Soreness and tenderness should be of short duration when the athlete is rested. If these problems persist, the athlete should see a physician. Adolescent girls and women participating in contact sports or in those in which the breasts come in contact with apparatus or equipment (e.g., fencing) should wear a properly fitted cup brassiere.

Any penetration wound to the breast or a cut or severe bruise to the nipple requires an EMS response and care rendered by a physician. The athlete may care for a simple bruise to the breast in the same manner as other bruises are treated.

Chest-Muscle Injury

The muscles of the chest may be injured as a result of throwing movements and certain types of swimming strokes, (e.g., the backstroke and butterfly). The resulting strain can

be cared for by applying ice and resting the athlete. Restricting upper-extremity movement will lead to quicker healing in the early stages of the injury. A simple sling and swathe (see pp. 117-118) worn during waking hours will help immobilize the extremity and hasten the healing process. Recovery will be dependent upon a thorough stretching and strengthening program for the shoulder musculature.

BACK INJURIES

Injuries to the back may involve the spine. If the athlete is unconscious, the assessment indicates possible spinal injury, or the mechanism of injury is forceful enough to produce spinal injury, you *must* assume that spinal injury has occurred. Injuries to the spine are discussed in chapter 12.

Remember that injury to the upper back may also involve internal chest injuries due to compression of the organs. Mid- and lower-back injury also may damage organs in the abdomen and pelvis, particularly the kidneys. Make certain that you consider these possibilities as you assess the injury.

Symptoms and Signs of Soft-Tissue Back Injury

When the soft tissues of the back are injured, the following symptoms and signs may be noted:

- *Pain.* This can be localized or may radiate out to the arms and legs. Most often, radiated pain will be down one or both legs and will increase with movement, though the athlete should not be asked to move to demonstrate this fact.
- *Restricted movement.* This results from muscle spasms and pain.
- *Muscle spasms.* These spasms may involve one or both sides of the back. When one side is injured, the athlete may lean in that direction.
- *Tenderness.* This may affect a large area of the back or may be limited to point tenderness.
- *Obvious open wounds or bruises.*

Care for Soft-Tissue Injuries to the Back

Many soft-tissue injuries to the back can be prevented by conditioning, teaching proper execution of skills, warm-ups that include stretching exercises, using the correct protective gear, and properly maintaining the playing field or surface, apparatus, and equipment.

Open Wounds

Open wounds to the back are cared for using the general wound care described in chapter 6. Be certain to assess the athlete for chest or abdominal involvement if there is a puncture wound to the back. The danger of pneumothorax does exist with deep penetrating back wounds.

Closed Wounds

Bruises to the back are common and most frequently result from falls or physical contact, with the highest incidence being reported in football. Most bruises to the back can be cared for by applying cold and compression; however, any bruise to the back that is the result of a forceful blow or serious fall *must* be evaluated by a physician. This is true even when there are no symptoms or signs that indicate possible spinal injury. Damage to the kidneys should be your primary concern. Only a physician can evaluate and determine the care of kidney injuries, including "bruised" kidneys. However, athletes should be alerted to look for signs of injury, including blood in the urine.

While the bruise is healing, the athlete should rest and refrain from activities that could result in another blow to the bruised area. This is especially important if the bruise is large since reinjury could lead to serious internal blood loss. If the bruise is located where it will be in contact with protective equipment, the injury site should be evaluated by a physician before the athlete is allowed to resume participation. In most cases, a custom-made pad will provide adequate protection of the bruised area. You should also evaluate the piece of protective equipment to determine why it did not prevent the original injury.

Back strain, especially to the lower back, is a common sport injury. Minor strain that is not associated with falls, contact, or sudden, force-ful twists can usually be cared for by rest. Most simple back strains are easily reinjured. The athlete must be rested until all symptoms and signs of the injury are no longer present. If the athlete is reinjured, he or she must see a physician no matter what the cause or where the reinjury occurred. Bent knee half sit-ups (curl-ups) done daily in conjunction with a stretching program prescribed by a physician will significantly reduce the chance of reinjury.

Regardless of the cause of a back injury, if the athlete has restricted movement of the trunk or extremities, any pain or restricted movement of the neck, pain or restricted movement of a limb, burning or tingling sensations or numbness, problems walking normally, or obvious pain, a physician's evaluation is necessary and an EMS response recommended.

ABDOMINAL INJURIES

Most abdominal injuries are mild: however, penetrating wounds and severe blows to the abdomen may cause a life-threatening injury. Because the abdominal cavity is rich with blood vessels, injury can produce profuse internal bleeding. In addition, the hollow organs of the abdominal cavity can be ruptured, releasing blood and digestive juices that can cause a severe reaction. Carefully assess the athlete's condition, looking for the symptoms and signs that will indicate the nature and severity of the injury. Be certain to look for related injuries to the chest, pelvis, and spine.

Symptoms and Signs of Abdominal Injury

Simple bruises, cuts, and scratches to the abdomen are usually obvious and tend to be minor. Assume that the injury is serious if you detect any of the following conditions:

- Changes in the level of consciousness. (Do not consider fainting or "passing out" to be a minor sign.)
- Severe pain. (If the athlete complains about the level of pain, shows facial expressions that indicate discomfort, or continues to hold his or her abdomen, consider the pain to be severe.)
- Pain that is at first mild and then becomes intolerable.

- Referred pain. (This is pain that occurs in body regions away from the injury site [see Figure 8.2]. The blow may be to the right side, but the pain may be more severe on the left. A blow to the liver and gallbladder may be indicated by pain over the right shoulder blade. Injury to the spleen may produce pain along the left side of the chest, the left shoulder, and the upper left arm.)
- Cramps.
- Indications of shock, especially weakness, nausea, thirst, rapid and shallow breathing, and a rapid and weak pulse.
- Puncture wounds.
- Large areas of bruises, an intense bruise, or a bruise of any size that is caused by a forceful impact.
- Coughing up or vomiting blood.
- Vomiting.
- A rigid and/or tender abdomen.
- Attempts by the athlete to guard his or her abdomen (he or she tries to lie very still and draws the knees up toward the chest).

Other signs may occur soon after the injury or could be delayed for several days. These signs include blood in the urine, dark stools (bleeding from the stomach or intestine), rectal bleeding, vomiting, and vomitus that contains substances that look like coffee grounds (partially digested blood). Instruct the athlete to look for these indications of possible injury. If the athlete is a minor, make certain that the parent or guardian is informed and instructed to look for these signs. Be sure to tell both the athlete and the parent or guardian that the athlete must see a physician as soon as possible if *any* of these signs appear. Let them know that these signs do not always mean that the injury is serious, only that the severity of injury *must* be determined by a physician.

Do not be mislead into thinking that the internal involvement of an injury is limited only to a particular area of the abdomen. A severe blow to one side of the abdomen can often cause damage on the opposite side. For example, a blow to the right side of the body can rupture the spleen, which is on the left side of the abdomen.

Care for Abdominal Injuries

Minor cuts and scratches can be cared for by using the general wound techniques described in chapter 6. In the event of abdominal injury, the athlete is usually most comfortable if placed

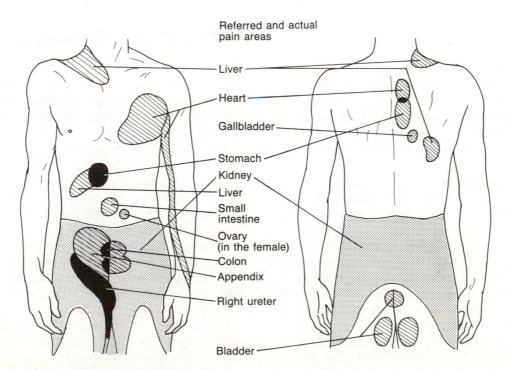

Figure 8.2. The patterns of abdominal pain.

on his or her back with the legs flexed at the knees. This will help relax the abdominal muscles and reduce pain.

Closed abdominal wounds can range from simple bruises to ruptured organs. Any of the symptoms and signs listed previously for possible severe abdominal injury must be considered when there is a closed abdominal injury. A simple bruise can be cared for by using a cold pack and compression, but remember that many serious internal injuries may at first be indicated by no more than a bruise.

Rest and monitor the athlete. Some athletes report greater comfort if they are allowed to hold a pillow or other soft, bulky object against the abdomen. Large bruises or those that result from a serious fall, contact, or impact require an EMS response.

Much has been written for coaches and trainers about bruised and ruptured organs. Bruised kidneys and livers and ruptured spleens do occur as a result of sport injuries, but as a coach you cannot diagnose them. A physician would not attempt to do a diagnosis without the athlete's history, a thorough exam, and the necessary tests. If the athlete shows any of the symptoms and signs of severe abdominal injury, assume that there is a serious problem and have someone alert the EMS system as you treat the athlete for shock.

Solar Plexus Injury

The solar plexus is located along the midline of the body just below the breastbone (see Figure 8.3). Blows to this nervous-system structure, even mild ones, may cause startling reactions. Some victims of blows to the solar plexus may experience a short period of unconsciousness. Other victims will have temporary problems with breathing (e.g., being unable to inhale). This type of injury is sometimes referred to as ''having the wind knocked out.''

If the athlete suffers a loss of consciousness, this may be a typical reaction to the injury; however, an EMS response is still necessary, as the loss of consciousness could signal numerous other more serious injuries. If an athlete has trouble breathing after a blow to the solar plexus, provide emotional support and ask him or her to relax. Have the athlete start a breathing pattern of a shallow inspiration followed by a long expiration. Loosen his

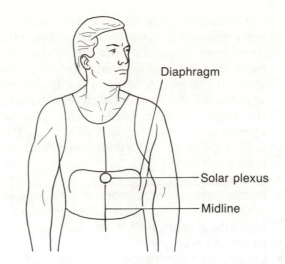

Figure 8.3. The location of the solar plexus.

or her belt and any clothing that is around the abdomen. Do *not* attempt to lift the trunk by pulling on the belt. This familiar practice is ineffective in helping the athlete breathe. Once the athlete is assured that he or she can breathe, have the athlete begin a normal pattern of breathing. With rest, the episode should pass quickly, but an EMS response is needed if the episode continues, there are symptoms or signs of other injury to the chest or abdomen, there is a loss of consciousness, or the force of the blow was severe.

''STITCH'' IN THE SIDE

A ''stitch'' in the side is a cramplike pain that occurs below the rib cage on the right or left side of the body. Some athletes experience referred pain at the shoulder. A stitch is typically seen as a chronic problem with poorly conditioned athletes who have an episode of this during or after running or a hard workout. Its cause is unknown, but there are indications that it often directly involves the diaphragm and the intercostal muscles (the muscles between the ribs).

You may find cases of a stitch that are probably related to poor breathing mechanics even in well-conditioned athletes. In these cases, add abdominal breathing exercises to the athletes' conditioning program.

Relief from a stitch can be brought about by having the athlete raise the arm on the same side as the stitch is on over his or her head and extend it as high as possible. If this procedure fails to relieve the cramps, the athlete should be directed to bend forward at the waist. These maneuvers and rest should bring quick relief. For cases in which the pain continues or increases, a health care professional or EMS response is recommended since the problem is probably more than a simple stitch. Continued problems with stitches, especially after improved conditioning, indicate that the athlete should be evaluated by a physician.

PELVIC AND GROIN INJURY

Soft-tissue injuries of the pelvic area present the same symptoms and signs as those of the abdomen. Remember that rectal bleeding and blood in the urine as well as bleeding from the urethra and vaginal bleeding associated with a trauma are signs of serious internal injury.

Hip Pointer

If you ask people to put their hands on their hips, most will place their hands over the upper part of the pelvis, an area called the *iliac crest*. A hip pointer is a bruise to this part of the body (see Figure 8.4). In some cases, the muscles may be severely bruised, but the most severe cases involve bruising the fibrous outer covering on the bones and/or fracturing

bones. In the growing athlete engaged in kicking sports, such as soccer, football, or rugby, one of the quadriceps muscles may be avulsed from its origin when the hip is extended and the knee flexed in the kicking motion. This injury is seen usually in contact sports when the iliac crest is not protected or is improperly protected, but it does occur frequently in football even when the proper protective gear is being worn. Volleyball players sustain hip pointers while diving for balls. Hip pointers are also possible from blows due to falls, striking apparatus or equipment, impact from hard balls (e.g., baseballs, golf balls, and lacrosse balls), or being struck by bats, sticks, or racquets. The typical hip pointer will produce pain and muscle spasms. The athlete must be rested, and cold and compression should be applied. Always be alert for the possibility of injury to the abdominal organs.

If the impact was forceful or if the hip pointer was produced as a result of a serious fall or striking a piece of apparatus or equipment, a health care professional or EMS response is necessary. If the athlete reports that he or she is unable to lift or flex the leg without experiencing pain or if he or she reports that trunk rotation is limited, an EMS response must be requested. These symptoms and signs must be viewed as being very serious since they also appear with hip fractures and dislocations (see p. 126). Do not request that the athlete attempt

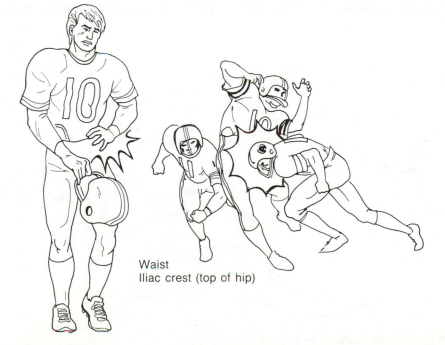

Waist
Iliac crest (top of hip)

Figure 8.4.   The hip pointer.

to move if he or she is lying down or in a semi-seated position.

When the athlete returns to action, he or she should wear a protective pad over the hip, especially if the athlete is involved in a contact sport. Watch for recurring trauma to the affected area.

Hernias

A hernia occurs when part of an abdominal or pelvic organ pushes its way through the abdominal wall. In males, this is most commonly seen in sports as an *inguinal hernia*, or "rupture." In most cases, the individual has a defect from birth that allows a portion of the abdominal membranes and perhaps the intestine to push through the inguinal canal. This is the opening through which blood vessels, nerves, and the cord from the testes pass. A forceful blow, a severe strain, an improper lifting technique, or an attempt to move weights while moving the legs apart or together (abduction and adduction, respectively) have been associated with hernias, though they are uncommon in young athletes. The *femoral hernia* occurs in females as membranes and the intestine are forced through the opening through which blood vessels and nerves run to the thigh.

In males, the bulging of abdominal structures into the scrotum may be felt or a protrusion seen. Pain and discomfort centered in the groin and abdomen accompany an inguinal hernia. Some inguinal hernias produce so much pain that the athlete faints.

The most dangerous condition is a strangulated inguinal hernia, which develops when the blood supply is cut off by the constriction of inguinal tissues (inguinal ring) around the protruding membranes and organ. This requires an EMS response and transport to a medical facility for surgery. Without surgery, the athlete may develop gangrene, which may lead to death.

The dangers of the strangulated inguinal hernia and tissue damage with the femoral hernia require the herniated athlete to be cared for by EMTs and transported to a medical facility. While waiting for the EMS response, you can help reduce the athlete's pain through proper positioning. It is usually best to let the athlete assume a position in which he or she feels most comfortable. You may suggest that the athlete try lying flat on his or her back with the body tilted head down at a 15° angle or face down with the knees resting against the chest (knee-chest position; see Figure 8.5).

The presence of a hernia does not necessarily disqualify an athlete for any sport. However, all inguinal and femoral hernias that lead to repeated episodes may require surgery at some point if the athlete wishes to continue participating in athletic activities. Athletic supporters, trusses, and exercises have not been shown to be effective in the healing or the prevention of recurring hernias.

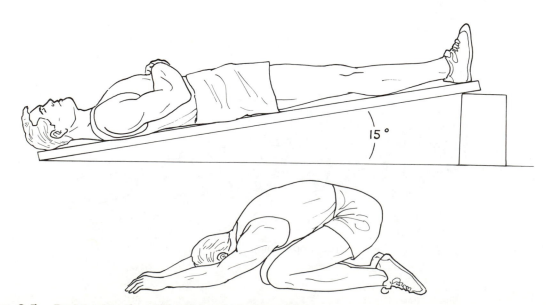

15°

Figure 8.5. Positioning the athlete to reduce hernial pain.

Groin Strains

The most common groin injury in sports is the groin strain, which involves the muscles of the inner thigh (adductor group). The strain is usually caused during running or jumping activities (e.g., football, volleyball, cheerleading, gymnastics), with the most serious injuries being associated with twisting forces. The athlete will report a sudden pain occurring during activity that increases after its onset. Stiffness in the groin, hip, or upper-leg muscles may occur.

Care for an athlete with groin strain includes immediate rest, cold packs, and compression. Several days or weeks away from participation will be required. Since a range-of-motion study and the assignment of stretching and progressive strengthening exercises is the best course of care, a physician's examination is recommended.

Injuries to the Genitalia

Injury as a result of contact to the external female genitalia is rare due to the protected location of the structures. Contact injury to the external male genitalia is more common and usually involves bruises to the scrotum and testes. Make certain that the athlete is given privacy for the interview and examination. You may also want to have an adult witness present for both questioning and any physical assessment. Explain what action you will be taking and why so that the athlete will feel more assured.

Closed wounds of the genitalia (bruises caused by forceful contact) can usually be treated with cold packs and light pressure. Some of the pain associated with bruises to the scrotum can be relieved by having the athlete lie on his back and pull his thigh to his chest. If any of the following occur to the male athlete at the time of injury or at any time after the injury, the athlete should report to a physician as soon as possible:

- Changes in the level of consciousness
- Swelling of the testes
- Swelling of the abdomen
- Swelling of the blood vessels in the scrotum, testes, or cord
- Continued dull pain and/or feelings of heaviness in the scrotum

- Sudden pain in the scrotum
- Nausea
- Vomiting
- Bleeding from the urethra

If the female athlete experiences any symptoms and signs other than mild pain due to a closed injury of the external genitalia, a health care professional or EMS response is necessary. Fainting must be considered to be a serious sign that requires immediate medical attention even when it is typical for the type of injury and pain produced.

SUMMARY AND RECOMMENDATIONS

A commonsense approach is called for when dealing with trunk injuries. In most cases, the injury will be a minor one that requires basic care and rest. In situations in which there are problems beyond mild pain or in which the forces causing the injury were severe, additional medical attention must be sought. Basically, the coach should never guess the nature of the problem or attempt a diagnosis. An error in assessment could be a serious mistake.

Keep these points in mind:

1. If function is impaired, a simple bruise can be cared for by applying a cold pack or compression and by resting the athlete. If function is not impaired, the athlete can apply a cold pack after the activity.
2. Simple cuts and scrapes can be cared for using basic wound-care procedures with the exception of an open wound of the nipple, for which the athlete should see a physician.
3. An open wound that has penetrated the chest cavity, breast, or abdomen requires an immediate EMS response.
4. Injury to the soft tissues of the back produce pain, restricted movement, muscle spasms, and tenderness. If a bruise is the result of a forceful blow or fall, assume that there may be a spinal injury or injury to internal organs.
5. Rest will correct most cases of back strain. If the strain is due to a fall, contact, or a sudden forceful twist, call for an EMS response. If the athlete

suffers reinjury after the strain heals, he or she *must* see a physician.

6. Most hip pointers can be cared for with rest, ice, and compression. However, those accompanied by limited movement or caused by forceful contact require medical evaluation.

7. Both males and females can experience hernias. Because of possible tissue damage and complications, the athlete should see a physician.

8. Groin strains can be cared for the same way as is any muscle strain, that is, with rest, ice, and compression.

9. Injuries to the external female genitalia are rare. However, if the athlete experiences severe pain or faints, medical assistance is required. The male athlete is more susceptible to genital injury. Be alert for signs of more serious internal injuries.

Chapter 9
Soft-Tissue Injuries—The Extremities

The soft tissues in the upper and lower limbs include skin, muscles, blood vessels, nerves, tendons, and ligaments. Tendons are strong cordlike elastic structures that attach muscles to bone, while ligaments are nonelastic fibrous tissue bands that connect bone to bone or bone to cartilage. The hard tissues of the extremities include bones and cartilage.

Most sport-related injuries to the soft tissues involve the skin and muscles; they usually are minor and can be easily cared for by applying the basic wound care presented in chapter 6. Cold and compression are effective in caring for most minor bruises. Basic dressing and bandaging techniques can be used for most minor cuts and scratches. When a joint is involved, special consideration must be given to the bandaging techniques to avoid cutting off circulation and binding the skin. The figure-eight bandage, as described on pages 68-69, helps to prevent these problems.

WARNING:

Compression and bandaging may interfere with circulation and nerve function. Always determine a distal pulse and assess for nerve function before and after rendering care for an injured athlete's extremity.

Sprains and strains are also frequent soft-tissue injuries. A *sprain* is actually a temporary, partial dislocation. The ligaments helping to support the joint are stretched and sometimes torn. The joint quickly realigns, almost immediately after the injury, so that the bone displacement commonly seen with dislocations is not present. A *strain* is commonly called a "pulled muscle." This injury involves the stretching and perhaps the tearing of muscle.

Field assessment of soft-tissue injuries is often difficult in the growing athlete because growth areas are often more vulnerable to stresses imposed by sports than are the ligaments and muscles. In more mature athletes, muscles are more prone to injury. As a result, it is difficult to determine whether an injury is a sprain, a strain, or a growth area injury by simply gathering a history of injury and evaluating what you have seen, felt, and heard. An X ray is required to make the appropriate diagnosis. Therefore, all possible sprains and most strains, especially those that interfere with function, should be cared for as if there were a fracture.

Although the official recommendation is to treat all sprains and strains as if they were fractures, often an experienced coach or trainer will determine that a minor strain or sprain has occurred and decide not to splint or call for an EMS response. However, if the apparent strain is related to a twisting injury, fall, impact, or contact or if there are any signs other than pain, do *not* assume that the injury is a minor one, particularly if the injury interferes with function. It is true that swelling and sometimes minor bruises are signs of sprains or strains, but they are also very strong indicators of more serious damage. Because of the similarity of sprains and strains to fractures, their care is discussed along with skeletal injury in chapter 10.

UPPER-EXTREMITY SOFT-TISSUE INJURY

The impacts, twisting forces, and repetitive motions associated with sports can lead to upper-extremity soft-tissue injuries. To ensure that a serious injury is not overlooked, the coach must consider the force causing the injury, the direction of the force, and the results of his or her assessment of the athlete. The assessment of an upper-extremity injury must include examining for possible fractures, dislocations, and disruption of circulation and nerve function.

The assessment for the disruption of circulation is done by checking for a radial pulse in the injured limb. A loss of nerve function is tested for by touching one of the athlete's fingers and asking the athlete if he or she can feel your touch. If there are no indications of a possible fracture or dislocation (deformity, rapid swelling, discoloration, or point tenderness), you can ask the athlete to wiggle his or her fingers and to grasp your hand. Any failure to perform these tests must be considered to be a sign of either compression on a nerve or a nerve or spinal injury.

Pulse and nerve assessment must be done before and after care is provided. If, for example, you bandage a wound and find that the radial pulse is no longer present, you must remove and reapply the bandage in case your bandaging procedure is responsible for the loss of the pulse. In any situation in which a lack of pulse or nerve function exists before care or is found after reattempting care, an EMS response is necessary.

The Shoulder Girdle

The shoulder girdle (see Figure 9.1) consists of the collarbone, or clavicle; the shoulder blade, or scapula; the joint made between the collarbone and the breastbone; the joint between the collarbone and the shoulder blade; the joint between the shoulder blade and the upper arm; and the soft tissues associated with these structures. Regardless of the nature of the injury to the shoulder girdle, you must consider the possibility of a fracture or dislocation and look for the symptoms and signs of these injuries in your assessment. The majority of injuries detected, however, will be less severe.

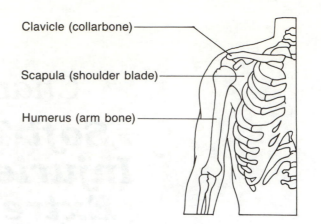

Figure 9.1. The shoulder girdle.

Bruises

Most bruises of the shoulder girdle result from impact in contact sports, falling on the tip of the shoulder, or being struck by a piece of apparatus or a hard ball. Pain is common and should be of low intensity. Temporary restriction of shoulder movement may be seen. The most painful bruise usually involves the lateral end of the collarbone where it joins with the shoulder blade. Rest, cold, and compression is the standard care. You should restrict the athlete from activities that could cause reinjury before healing is complete.

Inflamed Joint

Inflammation of a joint may have a sudden onset (acute injury) as a result of direct or indirect trauma or a gradual onset (chronic condition) from overuse of the weakened structures or from a repetitive action, such as throwing a ball. Acute conditions can become chronic ones if they are not allowed to heal properly or are not rehabilitated completely. Initial care for the inflamed joint, whether it be an acute or chronic injury, is RICE (rest, ice, compression, and elevation) and referral to a physician for evaluation. In the case of an acute injury resulting from direct impact or from pulling or twisting of the arm that may occur in sports such as football or wrestling, assume if the athlete has trouble moving the shoulder that a more serious injury exists. Immobilize the shoulder and arm with a sling and swathe (see pp. 117-118) and call for an EMS response.

Frozen shoulder, as the term implies, is a major limitation in shoulder movement and develops as the shoulder joints are inflamed over a long period of time. Typically, the athlete will have a history of shoulder pain, especially at night. In most cases, the limitation in shoulder movement will slowly become more pronounced. This is a very rare condition in the young athlete; therefore, never assume that this is the young athlete's problem. The joint should be immobilized and the athlete transported to a physician for evaluation.

The older athlete with a history of this problem should see a physician as soon as possible. If the problem can be related to an impact or to pulling or twisting of the arm, assume that there is a more serious problem, immobilize the joint and arm, and call for an EMS response.

Rotator-Cuff Injury

The rotator cuff consists of four deep muscles of the shoulder that connect the shoulder blade and the upper arm. Repetitive movements such as throwing a ball, swinging a racket, or swimming strokes (particularly the butterfly) may cause inflammation and pain in this area. This problem is seen in its most serious form in baseball pitchers and is perhaps due to overtraining or improper mechanics (not allowing the arm to follow through completely).

With overstress, the inflamed tendon and bursa are pinched by the overlying bone when the arm is moved away from the side of the body (abduction). Rest, cold packs, and compression should be provided. In addition, the injury must be evaluated by a physician. Typically a program to improve the strength and flexibility of each of the muscles of the rotator cuff is necessary to prevent reinjury.

Tears to the rotator cuff usually produce pain or reduced strength in moving the arm away from the midline of the body (abduction), in turning the arm outward (external rotation), or in turning the arm inward (internal rotation), depending on the muscles involved. Because it is not possible for the coach to assess this injury, any fall, twist, impact, or collision that produces long-lasting shoulder pain and restricted painful movement must be treated as a fracture or a dislocation.

Stingers

Force applied to the head, neck, shoulder, and sometimes the arm can mildly injure the nerves that run from the spine to the arm and produce a pain commonly called a *stinger*. Most stress is placed on these nerves when the head is forced to one side and, at the same time, the opposite shoulder is depressed. This type of injury is seen most often in football.

Immediately following impact, the athlete who is suffering a stinger will experience a momentary loss of function in the involved arm and shoulder (deltoid muscle). The athlete will have pain in the neck and shoulder as well as burning, tingling sensations that radiate down the arm. Numbness and tingling sensations in the fingers are common but should subside and disappear in 30-60 seconds. Function of the arm should return within a minute or two.

If the symptoms do not subside, you must assume that a more serious injury has occurred, keep the athlete lying still, and provide the same care as you would for a possible spinal injury (see pp. 136 and 137). If there is any indication that the numbness or tingling may be the result of a dislocated shoulder, carefully apply a sling and swathe (see p. 118). Even in these cases, the problem is usually a stinger, but you cannot guess or take the chance that treatment of a more serious injury will be delayed.

If the symptoms fade quickly, the athlete may return to activity unless he or she has experienced repeated cases of stingers. Athletes having recurring stingers must be rested and evaluated by a physician to determine if other problems are present.

The Upper Arm

Most upper-arm soft-tissue injuries are related to direct impact or repetitive movements. Serious injuries to the upper arm are sometimes followed by profuse internal bleeding or nerve damage. Do not delay medical care for any arm injury that you believe may be serious.

Bruises

Bruises are often seen in contact sports, with most occurring to the outside of the arm over the biceps muscle. Rest, cold packs with compression, and limited activity to avoid reinjury are recommended until healing is complete.

If the area is susceptible to repeated contact, a vinyl foam pad may be used to protect the area.

Biceps Tendinitis

This is an inflammation of the tendon that connects the long head of the biceps muscle to the shoulder blade. It is an overuse injury in which the muscle is not strong enough to withstand the demands placed on it and is often associated with baseball pitchers and tennis players (usually a result of the overhand motions required for successful performance). The athlete will have a continuous dull ache or pain at the front and medial portions of the shoulder, with irritation or tenderness found in the medial groove of the biceps where it enters the shoulder joint (see Figure 9.2). Even the slightest pressure with your fingertips may be very painful. The athlete's pain will usually increase when raising the affected arm away from the side of the body as in blocking a shot in basketball or rotating the arm outward as in the windup for a pitch in baseball. Even a simple, everyday activity such as putting on a jacket will be painful. With time, the athlete will feel a grating sensation in the biceps and may experience a weakening in grip strength.

This type of injury requires rest, the application of a cold pack with compression, and medical attention as soon as possible. Complete rest of the affected arm for about 2 weeks followed by reconditioning will be needed. If the symptoms and signs are related to a twisting, pulling, or falling injury or to direct contact, assume that a more serious injury exists. In such cases, immobilize the athlete's arm as you would for a fracture and alert the EMS dispatcher.

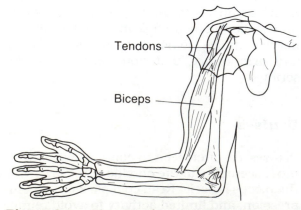

Figure 9.2.   The site of tenderness in biceps tendinitis.

The Elbow

The soft tissues of the elbow are usually injured by direct contact, repetitive movements, overexertion (such as "reaching back to put a little extra on the ball"), or improper mechanics. Bruises and joint inflammation of the elbow receive the same care as those of the shoulder. In the case of bruises of the posterior aspect of the elbow, it is recommended that an elbow pad be worn by the athlete even when the bruise appears to be healed, especially if the bursa (joint fluid sac) was irritated.

Whenever the elbow is forced beyond its normal straight alignment (hyperextension), you *must* assume that a dislocation or fracture has taken place and render the appropriate care. Usually a joint deformity will be present. Prior to the age of 13, children rarely suffer dislocations of this joint because of skeletal immaturity. For a child under 13, you may suspect a growth area injury.

When an athlete falls directly on his or her outstretched hand or shoulder and there are symptoms or signs of elbow involvement, you must assume that a fracture or dislocation is present and take appropriate action. Because of the likelihood of nerve and vascular trauma associated with a fracture or dislocation, check the pulse and coloration of nail beds. Also ask the athlete if he or she is experiencing any numbness or tingling sensations.

Elbow Inflammation—"Tennis Elbow"

As the name implies, this injury is most frequently a problem of tennis players and is often associated with the poorly conditioned "weekend player." For most tennis players, tennis elbow is caused by incorrect mechanics. Poor body position, court positioning, and timing will force the player to use only the arm on the backhand rather than stepping into the ball and transferring body weight "through the ball." The muscles on the outside of the elbow (the wrist extensors) are placed under considerable stress as they must absorb the impact of the ball on the tennis racket and impart force to the ball. The repeated stress leads to inflammation. A similar injury involving the lateral aspect of the elbow is also common to bowlers and golfers.

The athlete will usually complain of pain at the elbow that is not associated with an accident or a known injury. There will typically be a dull ache that radiates down the forearm. If allowed to go uncorrected, tennis elbow will develop as a chronic condition, grip strength will be reduced, and calcium deposits may form in the elbow.

Care requires rest and the application of cold and compression. A sling may be needed to restrict the player's use of the affected limb. Continued rest, a well-planned rehabilitation program, and instruction to correct improper mechanics are recommended. Chronic problems *must* be attended to by a physician. The danger of ligament calcification should not be taken lightly.

Elbow Inflammation—"Little League Elbow"

The medial aspect of the elbow can become inflamed due to the overhead motions produced in tennis and in pitching a baseball. Experienced tennis players sometimes develop this condition when they try to put too much spin on the ball. Inflammation is also directly related to throwing curving and breaking balls in baseball. With curve balls, incorrect technique is responsible for the inflammation, while the slider can cause inflammation even when the pitch is delivered correctly. We recommend that the use of these pitches be restricted to athletes in their late teens and older, when the growth area on the medial side of the elbow is closed. Adolescents should be limited in their use of this pitch. The care for this form of elbow inflammation is the same as for tennis elbow.

The Forearm

Most soft-tissue injuries to the forearm can be treated using the basic principles of wound care. Tendon inflammations should receive the same care as a significant bruise; however, the athlete should see a physician if the problem does not heal quickly.

The Wrist and Hand

Wrist injuries commonly result from falls on the hand, producing sprains, fractures, or dislocations (see chapter 11). Repetitive movements can also cause inflammations that should be cared for in the same manner as those produced in the elbow.

Bruises, cuts, and scrapes can be treated with general wound-care procedures. However, open injuries to the front (palm side) of the forearm and wrist are potentially dangerous because of the number of blood vessels located close to the body surface. What would be a mild puncture wound in another region of the body could produce serious bleeding from the distal forearm and wrist.

Wrist Ganglion

A wrist ganglion is a saclike structure filled with fluid that appears most frequently at the back of the wrist. The cause of a wrist ganglion is unknown, but the problem has been associated with joint-capsule and tendon inflammation, trauma, and repetitive motion. The ganglion is slow to heal but will usually disappear spontaneously. If the ganglion does not disappear, grows larger, or causes discomfort, the athlete must see a physician. Do *not* apply pressure to the ganglion or attempt to smash it. Not only do these procedures cause pain, but they may cause additional tissue damage and will neither rid the athlete of the ganglion nor improve the healing process. Ganglions have a tendency to recur regardless of the treatment prescribed.

Bruised Hand

Bruises to the back of the hand and the palm must be examined to rule out a possible fracture. Rest, ice, compression, and elevation should be used to provide initial care, with rest being essential. If the blow that caused the bruise was violent, it is best to assume that a fracture has occurred and immediately seek more highly trained assistance. If a treated bruise does not show positive signs of healing in 2-3 days, the athlete should see a physician. Padding may be required when the athlete returns to action.

Rips

Rips are tears to the surface of the palm and are usually associated with callus buildup or dry spots on the skin. They are most commonly seen as a problem of gymnasts and rowers, especially when palm guards or grips are not worn. Prevention is the best cure. Most rips can be prevented by filing the callus into a smooth surface and keeping the tissue soft and pliable. Warn your athletes not to file the callus so deeply that tender new skin is exposed. Simply remove the rough callus buildup and rub white petrolatum into the calluses every night.

Initial care for rips that do occur is the same as for any laceration: The athlete must rest to allow the wound to heal completely. Warn the athlete against using any steroid creams unless directed to do so by a physician as such medication promotes surface healing before deep healing, thus increasing the risk of recurring problems. If an athlete has repeated problems with rips, he or she should see a physician. Rip care during rehabilitation is discussed on page 209.

Injured Fingers

Soft-tissue injuries to the fingers that involve ligaments ("jammed" fingers) produce symptoms and signs that mimic fractures. Never try to realign a jammed finger by pulling on it as this may cause further damage to the soft-tissue structures. Instead, you should assume that a fracture has occurred, immobilize the affected part, and call for an EMS response. If the last segment of the finger is the only segment involved, splint the finger using a straight tongue depressor. Do *not* align the segment to splint. If either of the other segments is involved, you will need to immobilize the finger in a bent position by placing a roll of gauze or an elastic bandage in the palm of the hand.

Injuries to the fingertip may release blood under the fingernail (subungual hematoma), producing pain as pressure builds under the nail. Initial care requires a cold pack or soaking the injured digit in cool water for 10 minutes. The athlete will need to see a physician to have the pressure released. The doctor will bore a small hole in the nail to drain the blood.

If a nail is partially torn loose, do *not* remove the nail. The damaged nail can be used as a shield to protect the nail bed as new nail growth takes place. Dress and bandage the finger and have the athlete see a physician as soon as possible. A small portion of nail completely avulsed with no serious damage to the nail bed can be cared for with a simple dressing and bandage. The area will have to be cleaned, and the dressing should be changed frequently during the healing process. A commercial cage-type plastic fingertip guard can be applied to offer protection from additional injury. If the nail is fully avulsed or if there is any damage to the nail bed, dress and bandage the wound and arrange the appropriate transport to a physician. The damage may be more serious than is at first evident.

LOWER-EXTREMITY SOFT-TISSUE INJURIES

As in the case of soft-tissue injuries to the upper extremities, the coach must be certain that a fracture or dislocation is not part of the injury and that there is no serious damage to blood vessels or nerves. Once this is done, assessment of and care for soft-tissue injuries can begin, with a special effort being made to detect injuries that involve the soft tissues of the joints.

In any case that involves a blow or impact to the lower extremity, make certain that you monitor a distal pulse and check for distal nerve function both before and after care. Any disruption of pulse or lack of nerve function indicates a problem that requires immobilizing the injured limb (while protecting the spine) and calling for immediate medical attention.

The distal pulse that is used for the lower extremity is the posterior tibial pulse and is located behind the inner ankle. To test nerve function, touch one of the athlete's toes on the injured extremity. In most cases, this needs to be done without removing the athlete's shoe to avoid movements that could worsen fractures, dislocations, or nerve or spinal injuries. If there are no nerve or spinal injuries, the athlete should be able to tell you that he or she felt your touch.

The Thigh

The large muscle mass of the thigh is the site of many minor injuries. Unless the injured athlete is properly rested, reinjury is common. An athlete who is allowed to participate while suffering thigh pain may modify his or her movements to reduce the pain, which could result in knee, ankle, or hip injuries.

Bruises

Most bruises of the thigh result from impact in contact sports or from being struck by a piece of apparatus or a hard ball. The pain experienced by the athlete should be mild, and there should be no restriction in lower-extremity movement. If function is impaired, cold with compression and rest are the typical approaches to care. Restrict the athlete from activities that may allow reinjury before healing is complete. Padding will often prevent reinjury.

A deep bruise to the muscle group in the front of the thigh (quadriceps) is commonly called a *charley horse*. This type of injury produces a pocket of blood at the injury site that is called a *hematoma*. In addition to suffering pain, the athlete may experience minor swelling and some limitation in the outward rotation of the thigh, flexion of the hip, and contraction of the quadriceps.

There are two types of charley horse:

- A severe, or devastating, charley horse may keep the athlete from participating for an entire season.
- A mild, or nondevastating, charley horse usually has a short recovery period.

Once you are certain that the injury to the thigh is not anything more serious than a charley horse, bend the athlete's knee (without forcing it) to place a slight stretch on the muscles of the anterior thigh but not to the point of producing pain. Employ the RICE method (rest, ice, compression, elevation) to initiate care. While compression is being applied, have the athlete cross his or her hands and press on top of the injury site. This may help reduce internal bleeding.

After the final application of ice, wrap the thigh with a dry elastic wrap (see p. 207) to help control additional swelling. Be sure to wrap from the knee up toward the hip to prevent blood from pooling at the knee. Do not apply the wrap too tightly as this will restrict circulation in the limb. A vinyl foam pad that has been cut slightly larger than the tender area of the thigh can be placed under the wrap to spread the compression (see Figure 9.3). Have the athlete keep the knee bent to reduce muscle spasms and to maintain a slight tension, which will help improve the control of bleeding.

It is very important that the athlete who suffers a charley horse rests. Tell the athlete not to do anything that causes the muscle group to hurt. When possible, have the athlete use crutches for several days to restrict weight

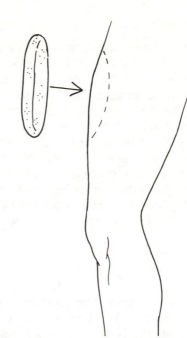

Figure 9.3. A vinyl pad applied to the injured area before bandaging can help spread the compression.

being placed on the injured limb, especially if he or she is limping.

After 24 hours, a physician or physical therapist should test the athlete's pain-free range of motion at the knee. This test will usually supply the information you need to determine how long the athlete will have to be rested, which can range from 1 week to the entire season.

Unlike other soft-tissue injuries where there is an option to start applying heat after 48 to 72 hours to promote healing, no heat should be applied to a charley horse while the athlete is recovering from the injury. In addition, the muscle group should not be massaged nor should the athlete attempt to stretch the tissue during this time. Applying heat or massaging the injured tissue too soon may disrupt the bruise (hematoma), delay healing, or lead to complications such as the growth of bone within the muscle (myositis ossificans). The hematoma should be completely absorbed before the athlete is allowed to return to activity.

The decision to return the athlete to activity should be that of the attending physician. A program of quadriceps stretching and strengthening directed by a physician should be completed before activity is allowed. A commercial or improvised vinyl pad should be worn by the athlete to help prevent reinjury.

Quadriceps Strain

The severity of a quadriceps strain can be determined by having the athlete lie face down on a table and bend the knee as far as possible without experiencing pain. You should compare this pain-free range of motion with that of the uninjured leg. If the athlete can bend the knee to a 90° angle or beyond, the strain is mild. If the knee cannot be bent to a 90° angle, the strain is moderate to severe. Pain may be felt as high as the pelvis because the most superficial (closest to the skin) of the quadriceps muscles crosses the hip joint as well as the knee.

You can check for severe tissue damage by feeling along the length of the muscle to detect "knots" or indentations in the muscle tissue. Always compare the injured with the uninjured sides. The immediate care for quadriceps strain is the same as that for a charley horse. Follow-up care should include a stretching and strengthening program.

Hamstring Strains

The posterior muscle group of the thigh is the hamstring group. All three of the hamstring muscles originate on the pelvis and connect to the lower-leg bones (either the tibia or the fibula). Muscle "pulls" to these muscles will usually produce pain that can be localized anywhere along the back of the thigh. Hamstring strains tend to recur, possibly because many hours of running and certain exercises tighten the hamstrings.

Once you are certain that the injury is not more serious than a "pulled" hamstring, have the athlete lie face down on a table and bend the knee to move the injured leg through its pain-free range of motion. You should compare this range of motion with that of the uninjured leg. Next, check for strength impairment. Place your hand on the athlete's calf and apply resistance as the athlete attempts to flex the knee (see Figure 9.4). Stop applying the resistance at the point of discomfort. If the athlete has a hamstring strain, there will be pain produced on resistance. The same thing will happen if the muscles are stretched in a sitting or semireclining position. The athlete will experience pain when he or she attempts a straight leg raise because the hamstring is stretched.

Hamstring strains, like other strains and sprains, may be mild, moderate, or severe. In the case of mild strain, the athlete may not feel any discomfort until after finishing the activity and cooling down. The athlete will usually recover completely in 3-7 days. With moderate strain, a loss of function will occur immediately. Recovery from this type of strain can be expected in 1-3 weeks. A severe strain or any hamstring strain that does not show steady healing may involve what is known as an *avulsion fracture*, which occurs when the muscle has pulled away (broken off) a piece of pelvic bone. All cases of severe hamstring strain or any hamstring strain that is not healing properly requires treatment by a physician. X ray analysis is usually necessary.

Youngsters participating in sports that require twisting and jumping (including cheerleaders)

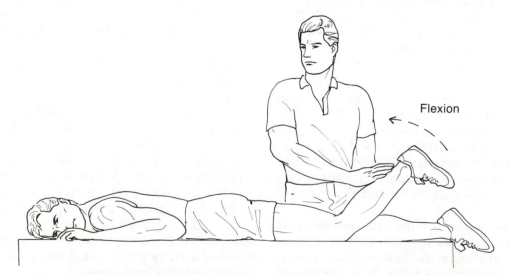

Flexion

Figure 9.4.   As a second step, apply resistance as the athlete flexes the injured leg.

may have one of the hamstring muscles tear away from the growth center of the pelvis. This condition can also occur in the medial (inner) thigh muscles known as the adductor group. If the individual has severe pain or is greatly restricted in the pain-free range when trying to flex the knee or pull the legs together, assume that a tear has taken place and treat the injury as a fracture.

A hamstring strain should be treated using the RICE method and a mild stretch of the muscles. After the last ice application, apply compression by placing a vinyl foam pad over the injury site and wrapping the thigh with an elastic bandage starting at the knee and finishing at the upper thigh (p. 207). Stress on the hamstrings can be reduced by placing a heel lift in the shoe.

Thigh-Muscle Cramps or Protective Spasms

These cramps are the painful contractions of one or more of the thigh muscles and are usually caused by fatigue, by water loss, or by inadequate stretching, conditioning, and warm-up. In some cases, overexposure to cold or poor circulation may cause the onset of leg-muscle cramps. Any one of these factors may activate a cycle of increasing muscle tightness. Such cramps or spasms also occur in calf and abdominal muscles.

Most thigh-muscle cramps can be relieved by stretching the muscle, which will "turn off" the nerve that is responsible for the cramp. For example, the quadriceps at the front of the thigh can be stretched by bending the knee (only to the point of discomfort). The muscles should be held on stretch for about 1 minute and then slowly released. If the muscle tightens, it should be stretched again cautiously.

If poor circulation is the possible cause of muscle cramps, have the athlete consult a physician. Immediate care requires the muscle to be massaged while being stretched using a gentle rubbing action toward the heart. Avoid any motion that will knead the muscle. The massage will help stimulate the circulation in the affected area.

The body puts a muscle in a spasm as a protective mechanism. In a sense, the body is "splinting" injured or damaged tissues. Whenever a cramped muscle does not respond to stretching, massage, and/or fluid replacement, assume that some tissue has been damaged.

Treat the injury site with the RICE method plus stretching and refer the athlete to a physician.

The Knee

The soft tissues of the knee can be injured as a result of impact, twisting forces, improper conditioning, poor equipment, or poor playing surfaces. Great care must be taken to be certain of the nature of the knee injury and its possible extent. When in doubt, assume that the injury is very serious and provide care as if one of the bones making up the knee were fractured. Dislocations and fractures of the knee will be discussed in chapter 11.

Overstress Injury

A common overstress injury of the knee involves the cartilage on the back of the kneecap (patella). The medical term for this injury is *chondromalacia patellae*, which means the softening of the cartilage of the kneecap.

Overstress injury is usually not the direct result of a single trauma or impact to the knee. If pain is reported after a knee injury, it is probably due to another cause. Overstress injury is progressive. Wear on the surface of the posterior cartilage is typically minor at first and becomes more pronounced with time. The kneecap will no longer slide smoothly along the lower surface of the thigh bone. The cartilage behind the kneecap will soften and continue to wear away. The athlete will complain of a persistent pain behind the kneecap, present when sitting, walking, or climbing and descending stairs and will experience a painful grating sensation when the knee is moved. In most cases, the underside of the inner edge of the kneecap will also be tender.

Any athlete with indications of an overstress injury of the knee must see a physician. Do not allow the athlete to use stairs or keep the knee constantly bent or straightened. Arrange a slow, progressive rehabilitation program after consulting the attending physician. Do not allow the athlete to do flexion/extension exercises that involve the knee unless directed to do so by a physician.

Jumper's Knee

Jumping should be viewed as an explosive act that places enormous stress on the anterior thigh muscles, especially along the tendons of insertion for the quadriceps muscle group. Athletes who compete in sports that require much jumping may develop jumper's knee, which is a form of tendinitis that requires the attention of a physician. The indications of jumper's knee include the following:

- Localized pain where the tendon joins the kneecap, either above or below the kneecap
- Aching and stiffness following inactivity

Osgood-Schlatter's Disease

This condition involves the bony projection just below the kneecap (the tibial tubercle), the site of insertion for the quadriceps. The disease is seen most frequently in young male athletes between the ages of 10 and 15; however, the emergence of more young females in competitive athletics is causing the incidence among that sex to increase.

This condition is not associated with a single impact or any other form of trauma but is caused by the inflammation of the quadriceps tendon or the separation of the growth center (both due to poor circulation) where the muscle group is attached. The problem is most often associated with poorly supervised weight-training programs in which the knee is bent too much (hyperflexed) and heavy weights are being lifted.

The athlete will typically experience pain at the bony projection below the kneecap and may begin to limp. The area below the kneecap is tender and kneeling painful. Although the problem tends to be self-limiting, the athlete should be examined by a physician. Inactivity may be necessary for healing to take place. Consult with the attending physician to develop a program of quadriceps stretching and strenghtening. The area around the sensitive bony projection should be padded whenever the athlete is active.

Prepatellar Bursitis

A *bursa* is a fluid-filled sac that lies between moving tissues in a joint, and *bursitis* is an inflammation of a bursa. The prepatellar bursa lies directly on top of the kneecap between the bone and the skin. A severe blow or repeated blows to the kneecap may break blood vessels in the sac and cause the lining of the bursa to

secrete an overabundance of fluid, leading to the swelling of the sac.

This is a common injury in volleyball, basketball, gymnastics, and other sports in which athletes frequently fall on their knees. If there is any doubt about the nature of the injury, assume that the athlete has a fractured kneecap.

Initial care requires applying ice and then using an elastic bandage to reduce pain and swelling. To allow compression to be evenly applied over the affected area, cut a vinyl foam pad into the shape of a horseshoe to fit around the bottom edge of the kneecap before applying the elastic bandage (see Figure 9.5). Once the bursa is healed, have the athlete wear a knee pad to help prevent reinjury. If the pain and swelling do not diminish or if additional range of motion is lost, have the athlete treated by a physician.

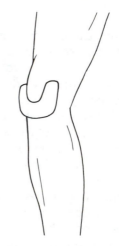

Figure 9.5. Use a vinyl horseshoe to spread compression evenly in treating prepatellar bursitis.

Water on the Knee

Water on the knee is called *synovitis* and is an inflammation of the lining of the fibrous capsule, the synovial membrane, that surrounds the joint. Whenever the synovial membrane is irritated, regardless of the cause, an abnormal amount of lubricating fluid is produced, which causes swelling to occur within the joint cavity.

The swelling caused by injury to the bursa over the top of the knee will cause swelling on top of the kneecap. Injury to the synovial lining will produce swelling inside the capsule, underneath the kneecap.

Any athlete with water on the knee must see a physician. Swelling that takes place immediately after a blow or other form of trauma to the knee must be treated as a fracture, and an EMS response must be requested.

The Lower Leg

Simple bruises to the lower leg can be cared for by using the RICE method. There are, however, several other types of lower-leg injuries that you should be prepared to care for. If an athlete complains of lower-leg pain immediately after a hard, direct blow to the lower leg (e.g., a football helmet striking the lower leg during a tackle), twisting forces applied to the leg, or a fall in which the athlete lands on his or her foot, and function is impaired, then consider the injury to be serious and treat the leg as if there were a fracture.

Calf Strain

Strain to the lower leg can occur anywhere along the muscles from the lower thigh to their insertions on the heel. If the primary calf muscle (the gastrocnemius) is strained enough to produce pain and protective muscle spasms that decrease the athlete's range of motion, restricting activity will be necessary until the normal pain-free range of motion is regained. If the pain is severe, the athlete will need to be seen by a physician.

Many cases of calf strain produce severe pain, interfere with the ability to walk without a limp, and require the athlete to use crutches during the initial stages of healing. For less serious strains, place a heel lift in the shoe to restrict the foot's range of motion and thus reduce stress on the injured calf muscle. Once the range of motion is normal, assign the athlete to a rehabilitation program that will strengthen and stretch the calf muscle. (More information on rehabilitation programs is included in chapter 16.) The rehabilitation of serious strains will have to be carried out under the direction of a physician.

Shin Splints

"Shin splints" is the common name given to an overstress muscle injury in the lower leg. If the stress of an activity is greater than the muscle's strength to withstand that stress, a muscle strain may occur. When this happens, the athlete will feel a pain in the muscle mass in the lower leg along either the outside border of the shin (tibia) or the lower inside border of the shin. Unless steps are taken to alleviate this condition when the athlete first complains, repeated stress may cause the inflammation of other structures in the lower leg.

The onset of shin splints should be taken as a serious warning. As the muscles pull on their attachments, the membrane between the two lower-leg bones (the interosseous membrane) may be subjected to overstress. This membrane may eventually stretch and could possibly tear. Continued stress may cause the muscles to pull away from the outer fibrous covering of the bone (periosteum).

You must learn to recognize the symptoms of shin splints on the basis of what the athlete tells you about pain during activity. Always take the athlete out of the activity the moment that the first discomfort in the shin is felt. Since other people may give the athlete incorrect information, be sure to tell the athlete that shin splints cannot be "run out."

When the athlete complains of shin splints, you must try to identify the contributing factors causing the injury. Some of the causes include arch weakness, muscle imbalance, improperly fitted shoes, and continued pounding on hard surfaces. One of the primary causes, however, is incorrect running mechanics. Always watch for foot placement when an athlete runs: He or she should *not* run on the toes. In distance running, the athlete should land on the heel, roll off along the outer border to the ball of the foot, and push off. Slapping the toes down or toeing out while running increases the stress on the lower-leg muscles.

Once incorrect running mechanics are discovered, you should teach the athlete to run with the toes pointed straight ahead or slightly inward. This can be done by having the athlete run along a straight line. Slapping the foot can be controlled by strengthening the front muscles of the lower leg. When you instruct the athlete in the proper mechanics of running, remember to be patient since it is more difficult to change form than it is to gain muscular strength.

Improper conditioning and warm-up programs may cause a strength imbalance between the front and back lower-leg muscles, thus contributing to the shin splints. An imbalance may occur if exercises for the lower leg focus on strengthening only the calf muscles. Overstress injuries can be greatly reduced by using correct conditioning and warm-ups. Your early-season training program should also include exercises that will strengthen the muscles on the front of the lower leg and in the arch of the foot. This is necessary since the muscles that support the arch originate on the lower leg.

In some cases, shin splints may be caused by a too-rigorous training schedule. You should check your schedules to see if you have planned too much activity too early in the season. If several athletes begin to develop pain in the lower leg, reduce the intensity of the training activity.

Another problem to be considered regarding the development of shin splints is your program of early-season running. Your running program must ensure that shoes are properly fitted and broken in; running is on a well-maintained, smooth surface (a track when possible); the running of laps is alternated clockwise and then counterclockwise; there is a strengthening program for the lower legs; and stretching exercises for the muscles at the front and the back of the lower leg are included in the daily warm-up.

Exercises for strengthening the lower-leg muscles can be assigned. Additional information can be found in the ACEP Level 2 Sport Physiology Course described at the front of this book. The program that you use should focus on the manual resistance-to-range of motion exercises. Stretching exercises for the calf muscles are also necessary since they tend to tighten with repetitive running.

WARNING:

If an athlete reports experiencing continuous pain on the front or outside of the leg while at rest, restriction of movement in the toes or foot, numbness or coldness in the toes or foot, or any other complications after leaving the athletic arena, he or she should be instructed to call for EMS transport. These could be signs of more serious injuries, including a lower leg fracture or compartment syndrome.

Stress Fracture

This type of injury may mimic the onset of shin splints. You should suspect a stress frac-

ture of the tibia if, after a repetitive activity, the athlete experiences tenderness on the inside of the lower leg, usually 2-4 inches below the line of the knee joint or between the middle and lower thirds of the bone shaft. Stress fractures of the fibula, the non-weight-bearing bone on the outside of the leg, usually occur in the lower third. In either case, tenderness will be well localized (i.e., it could be covered by a fifty-cent piece). The pain will typically continue for several days without diminishing. When this occurs, be sure the athlete is examined by a physician. If this localized tenderness occurs immediately after impact, treat the injury as if there were a fracture.

The Ankle

Many injuries to the ankle are possible. Sprains, perhaps the most common, can be treated using the RICE method. Additional discussion of sprains is included in chapter 11.

Soft-tissue injuries to the ankle that involve the Achilles tendon often become chronic problems unless time is given for proper healing. At the first sign of recurring problems, rest the athlete.

Achilles Tendon Strain

A simple strain to the Achilles tendon is common in many sports. The athlete will usually report pain and a feeling of weakness above the heel when trying to move the foot. Care must be taken in evaluating the injury so that possible sprains and fractures are not overlooked. The RICE method can be used as the initial care procedure for this type of strain. After the last 30-minute cold application (swelling has subsided and major internal bleeding is controlled), a dry elastic bandage can be applied using a figure-eight wrap (pp. 203-204) to help reduce swelling. The elastic bandage should not be applied too tightly since swelling may be delayed. Heel lifts should be placed in both shoes to reduce the stretch placed on the injured tendon and to prevent stress on the back due to unequal leg length when only one lift is worn. Rest the athlete until the injury is fully healed. Full recovery is dependent on a thorough stretching and strengthening program.

If the injury does not heal quickly (in a few days) or if swelling, pain, or weakness increases, have the athlete seen by a physician. If the signs of the injury are more serious, there is loss of function, or the athlete complains of a snapping sensation at the moment of trauma, treat the injury as you would a fracture, using a soft splint (see pp. 129-130).

Ankle Inflammation

As with other movable joints, inflammation of the ankle can be acute or chronic. The majority of acute injuries are mild to moderate sprains in which the sole of the foot is turned inward (inversion sprain). This is a common occurrence in basketball following a rebound, when a player comes down on another player's foot and the ankle turns due to the uneven landing.

Overstress injuries—tendinitis of any muscle crossing the joint or bursitis—make up the majority of chronic injuries seen in the ankle. In addition, an improperly rehabilitated ankle sprain leads to an unstable ankle that can be reinjured by merely stepping on a crack in the sidewalk.

Acute injuries that affect function and all overstress injuries should be evaluated by a physician. Initial care for both will require rest, ice, compression, and elevation. Later, with the permission of the physician, you should start a rehabilitation program to reduce the probability of the injury recurring.

The Foot

Anatomical problems of the foot, such as overlapping toes or chronic arch strain, among others, should be evaluated by a physician. Follow the physician's guidelines to help prevent injury or reinjury. Minor fractures and stress fractures may go undetected immediately following injury. Continued pain, tenderness, swelling, discoloration, or any loss of function requires that the athlete be seen by a physician.

Heel Bruise

This type of injury can be very painful and will usually limit the athlete's participation. Proper healing is necessary to help prevent reinjury. The most significant part of care is getting immediate rest, keeping weight off the injury site, and applying ice. The athlete should be instructed not to put weight on the heel for *at least 24 hours*. A heel cup with a vinyl foam heel pad is recommended once the athlete becomes active. The heel pad should have a cut-out area that corresponds to the size and location of the bruise.

Arch Strain

Factors that can lead to arch strain include poor conditioning, wearing the wrong type of shoes or improperly fitted ones, being overweight, excessive participation, and preexisting problems with the arch. The athlete will usually complain of weakness or tiredness, and a spot on the arch may be tender to the touch. Pain may occur anywhere along the arch from the ball of the foot to the heel. Arch strain is best cared for by resting the athlete and providing a therapeutic program to recondition the muscles of the foot and lower leg that support the arch.

SKIN PROBLEMS

Most sport-related skin problems of the extremities consist of minor injuries to the hands or feet. Whenever a minor injury does not show improvement or the problem worsens with care, the athlete must see a physician.

Blisters

Blisters are soft-tissue injuries that are friction burns. A layer of skin is separated from underlying tissues, which allows fluid to collect in the resulting space. Capillary bleeding between the layers may also occur. Blisters are caused by repeated rubbing or pinching of the skin and are most frequently formed on the feet due to sudden stops and starts and changes of direction and of speed.

The coach's approach to blisters should be one of prevention. The best approach to controlling blister formation on the feet is to have your athletes wear the proper shoes for the activity. These shoes must fit properly and be well broken in. New shoes should be broken in slowly, initially being worn only 5-10 minutes of each practice. If rough spots in the shoes such as stitching or eyelets cause irritation, the affected areas on the foot should be padded. Use a gauze pad set over a thin layer of lubricant such as petroleum jelly. If the skin is irritated, use a mild antiseptic cream under a sterile gauze or moleskin pad and tape the pad securely in place. Finally, blisters can be prevented by filing all callused areas so they are smooth.

Make sure that your athletes wear at least one pair of socks. Cotton or wool are preferable to most synthetic fibers because they are absorbent. There must be sufficient elasticity in the cuffs to keep the socks from sliding down to form blister-producing wrinkles. Instruct your athletes to change their socks daily. All socks must be washed prior to use. If the standard sock seams irritate the foot, tube socks can be worn or the socks can be worn inside out.

If the athlete has an unbroken blister, *do not puncture it*. Leave the blister unbroken and take the following steps:

1. Clean the area with mild soap and warm water.
2. Spread a thin coating of lubricant over the top of the blister.
3. Cover the site with several sterile gauze pads and paint the surrounding area with liquid tape adherent (if available).
4. After the adherent dries, tape the pads securely in place with clear plastic tape (which reduces friction) or athletic tape.

The dressing must be removed after practice or play and the site cleaned. A fresh dressing should be applied without lubricant. The injured area should be kept padded even after the blister has healed.

If the blister is open, you should care for it in the following manner:

1. Clean the area with mild soap and warm water.
2. Trim the torn edges of the blister using forceps (tweezers) and scissors that have been soaked in isopropyl alcohol.
3. Cut a "horseshoe" out of a piece of ¼-inch felt padding or moleskin so that the "horseshoe" is slightly larger than the blister.
4. Paint the area around the blister with liquid tape adherent and allow this to dry. Place the horseshoe so that it surrounds the blister. It is important that you avoid applying tape adherent to the blister as this not only will be painful

but will cause the blister to dry out too quickly and hinder healing.
5. Apply a small amount of water-soluble antiseptic cream in the horseshoe opening, cover the site with a sterile gauze pad, and, tape the pad in place.

After activity, remove the dressing and clean the injury site and surrounding area. Apply a very thin layer of antiseptic cream (just enough to cut down friction). Cover the affected area with several gauze pads and hold them in place with a gauze roller bandage, which can be held more securely if it is taped in place. Do not apply the tape directly over the blister. This same procedure can also be used for unbroken blisters.

The care for an open blister must be continued until the blister is fully healed. Protect the affected area with a horseshoe pad during practice but discontinue the protection after activity. Instruct the athlete to apply a thin layer of lubricant to the area at night to keep the skin pliable.

Encourage athletes who are prone to developing blisters to apply a lubricant to the problem areas. Have your athletes become aware of any "hot spots" that develop during practice. Have a pan of ice water, towels, and some lubricant near the sidelines ready for use. Tell the athlete who develops a hot spot to soak this area until it is numb, dry the area thoroughly, and apply a lubricant before returning to the activity. If hot-spot areas are cooled off right away, blistering can be prevented. Ice-water soakings should not be done outdoors in cold weather.

Blisters are often considered minor injuries. However, don't be lulled into failure to provide adequate care. Persistent blisters, corns, and calluses should be evaluated by a physician.

Calluses

A callus is a mass of dead skin tissue that builds up because of continual irritation. Some callus formation occurs naturally at weight-bearing points such as the edge of the heel, the edges of the first and fifth toes, and the balls of the feet. This natural, light callus formation is desirable. Excessive, hard-callus formation can lead to blisters as the rough tissue is rubbed back and forth creating friction. If calluses are allowed to remain, their buildup leads to cracking and splitting and invites skin infection.

To remove excess callus buildup, soak the callused area in warm, soapy water to make the skin more pliable. After drying, the callus may be filed down and smoothed with an emery board, callus file, or pumice stone. Once most of the callus is removed, the skin may be softened with daily applications of lubricant or pure lanolin.

Corns

Corns are caused primarily by tight-fitting shoes. Hard corns are the result of pressure and friction, while soft corns tend to form where there is friction and excessive perspiration (e.g., between the fourth and the fifth toes). Problems with hard corns can be treated best by taking pressure off the site using a felt doughnut or horseshoe pad. Soft corns should be washed daily in mild soap and water and dried thoroughly. After drying, a small piece of lamb's wool can be inserted between the adjacent and often overriding toes to dry moisture while allowing air to circulate between the toes. The lamb's wool should be replaced before it becomes saturated with moisture. A nonmedicated powder can be placed in the athlete's socks to help absorb perspiration. If a corn must be removed, have the procedure done by a physician. Commercial corn-removal preparations are not recommended because some contain ingredients that may damage healthy skin.

SUMMARY AND RECOMMENDATIONS

Most sport-related injuries to the soft tissues of the extremities can be cared for by applying basic wound-care procedures.

1. Minor cuts and scratches can be treated using dressings and bandages.
2. Cold and compression is usually all that is needed for minor bruises. Rest followed by limited activity and a sensible rehabilitation program is all that is needed to ensure good healing.
3. Specific extremity care is reviewed in Table 9.1 on page 110.

Table 9.1
Specific Care of Soft-Tissue Injuries to the Extremities

Injury	Care
Upper Extremities	
Inflamed shoulder joint	Cold, compression, rest
"Frozen shoulder"	Immobilization, EMS response
Rotator-cuff injury	Cold, compression, rest, and evaluation by a physician
Rotator-cuff injury (possible tear)	Treat as a fracture or dislocation
Biceps inflammation (tendinitis)	Cold, compression, and evaluation by a physician
Ruptured biceps	Treat as a fracture
Hyperextended elbow	Assume a fracture or dislocation and treat as a fracture
"Tennis elbow"	Cold, compression, rest; use a sling to restrict movement; instruct athlete in proper mechanics of play; have chronic problem cases seen by a physician
Elbow inflammation	Same as "tennis elbow"
Wrist ganglion	Self-correcting; if chronic, evaluation by a physician
Bruised hand	Cold, compression, rest; if cause by violent trauma, treat as a fracture
Injured fingers	When in doubt, treat as a fracture
Blood under fingernail	Cold therapy, drainage to be done by a physician
Torn fingernail	Small portion: dress and bandage; Large area: dress, bandage, have seen by a physician; Fully avulsed: dress, bandage, EMS transport to see a physician
Lower Extremities	
Bruised thigh	Cold, compression, rest, padding to prevent reinjury

Injury	Care
Charley horse	Flex knee to evaluate severity, RICE method, athlete applies hand compressions, dry elastic bandage wrap, re-evaluate after 24 hours, apply heat after 72 hours
Quadriceps strain	Evaluate knee flexion, treat initially as a charley horse
Hamstring strain	Evaluate knee flexion with resistance, RICE method and mild stretch, pad and elastic bandage wrap, heel lift
Groin strain	See chapter 8
Thigh-muscle cramps and spasms	Stretching, massage, RICE and stretch
Overstress injury (knee)	See a physician
Jumper's knee	See a physician
Osgood Schlatter's Disease	See a physician, rest, quadriceps stretching and strengthening
Prepatellar bursitis	Cold, horseshoe pad and elastic wrap, rest, pad to prevent reinjury
Water on the knee	See a physicians; if immediately after impact, treat as a fracture
Calf strain	Rest (crutches if needed), heel lift, rehabilitation
Compartment syndrome	Treat as a fracture
Shin splints	Immediate rest, correct contributing factors
Stress fractures	Treat as a fracture
Achilles tendon strain	RICE method, dry elastic bandage, heat therapy after 72 hours, heel lifts
Ankle inflammation	Immediately after impact: see a physician; slow to develop: rest, heat therapy, heel lifts, cold therapy after activity
Heel bruise	Rest, keep weight off site, heel cup or taping
Arch strain	Rest and therapeutic program

Chapter 10
Basic Principles of Skeletal Injury Care

The immediate detection of possible skeletal system injuries is very important as a slight delay in detection could lead to severe damage to blood vessels, nerves, and other soft tissues. Even when the coach does not splint the injury, detecting these skeletal injuries and keeping the athlete at rest are important parts of the care process.

For bone and soft-tissue injuries to follow a desired course of healing, the injured limb should be immobilized as soon as possible. This is especially true in the cases of children and adolescents, who still have significant bone growth and development taking place. At the ends of the bones in the arms and legs are growth plates, or areas of active elongation and growth. Damage to these growth plates (epiphyseal plates) is a serious injury that can affect growth in the involved extremity. Vascular and neural complications may accompany trauma to the bones in skeletally immature athletes.

In most cases, the EMS or health care professional who is responding should arrive soon enough after a skeletal injury so that the coach will not have to splint the injured limb. The coach instead can concentrate on controlling bleeding, dressing serious open wounds, and beginning the care for shock. During such care, the athlete should not be moved, nor should the injured limb be lifted or repositioned. Splinting should be done by the coach only when properly trained and certified to do so, when a professional response is delayed, and when splinting is expected to be done by the coach according to local policy. If you are required by local policy to splint, review the procedures very carefully.

THE SKELETAL SYSTEM

All the bones and their joints form the skeletal system, which is involved with support, protection, and movement. Tissues inside some bones are involved in blood-cell production. Bones are living tissues supplied with blood vessels and nerves.

There are two major divisions of the skeletal system: the *axial skeleton* and the *appendicular skeleton*. The axial skeleton is the upright axis of the body and consists of the skull, spine, breastbone, and ribs. The appendicular skeleton is the upper and lower extremities. The pelvis is part of the lower extremity.

The upper extremity is composed of the following bones (see Figure 10.1):

- Collarbone, or clavicle
- Shoulder blade, or scapula (The shoulder blade and collarbone form the shoulder, or pectoral girdle.)
- Arm bone, or humerus (extends from the shoulder to the elbow)
- Medial (inner or little finger side) forearm bone, or ulna
- Lateral (outer or thumb side) forearm bone, or radius
- Wrist bones, or carpals (eight per wrist)
- Hand bones, or metacarpals (five per palm)
- Finger bones, or phalanges (14 per hand)

The lower extremity begins with the pelvis and consists of the following structures (see Figure 10.2):

- Thighbone, or femur (The pelvis and hips form the pelvic girdle. The hip joint is the

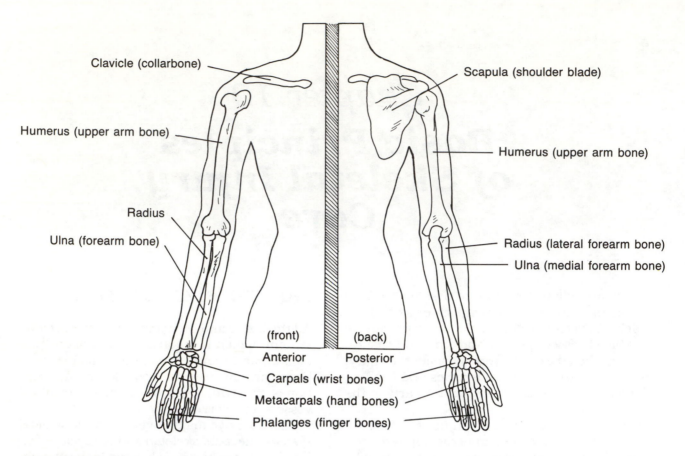

Figure 10.1. The upper extremity.

ball-and-socket joint where the thighbone joins the pelvis.)
- Kneecap, or patella
- Medial (inner) leg bone, or tibia
- Lateral (outer) leg bone, or fibula
- Ankle bones, or tarsals (seven per foot)
- Foot bones, or metatarsals (five per foot)
- Toe bones, or phalanges (14-15 per foot. Some persons have two little-toe bones; others have three.)

BONE AND JOINT INJURIES

Common injuries to the bones and joints include fractures, dislocations, and sprains. It is often difficult to tell which has occurred or whether two or more of the injuries exist at once. For example, an athlete may have a dislocated ankle with fractures to one or more of the bones that form the joint. In some cases, as when the cause of the injury indicates a likely fracture or when the symptoms and signs are not clear, it is wise to assume that the injury is a possible fracture.

Fractures

A fracture occurs whenever a bone is cracked, chipped, or broken. There are two major types of fractures:

- *Closed fracture.* This consists of damage to the bone and surrounding soft tissues, but the skin is not broken. The old term for this type of fracture is a *simple fracture.*
- *Open fracture.* This consists of damage to the bone and to surrounding soft tissues, and the skin is broken. The skin may be torn open by the ends or the pieces of bone, or the skin damage may be due to an object penetrating the body and fracturing a bone. The old term for this type of fracture is a *compound fracture.*

There is a third term that is often used in the emergency care classification of fractures. This is an *angulated fracture* and occurs when the fractured bone or joint takes on an unnatural shape. For example, the long bone of the upper arm may be broken in half to form

Anterior view

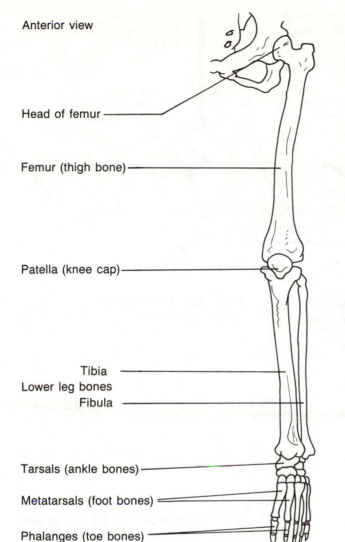

Head of femur

Femur (thigh bone)

Patella (knee cap)

Tibia
Lower leg bones
Fibula

Tarsals (ankle bones)

Metatarsals (foot bones)

Phalanges (toe bones)

Figure 10.2. The lower extremity.

a bend between the shoulder and the elbow. Many closed and some open angulated fractures can be straightened by emergency medical personnel; however, this requires specialized training. You should refrain from repositioning the limbs unless you have such training.

Finally, there are two types of fractures seen only in skeletally immature individuals. The first type involves the growth plates. There are actually three different growth plate injuries: physeal separations, epiphyseal separations, and apophyseal separations.

The *physis* is the actual growth plate, an area of cartilage close to the end of the bone where growth in bone length takes place. This area may be damaged by either a direct blow or a twisting motion.

The *epiphysis* is located at the end of a long bone and includes the smooth cartilage that lines the bone ends. It is separated from the shaft of the bone or diaphysis by the growth plate (physis).

The *apophysis* is a growth center that is part of a muscle attachment. In children and adolescents it is not uncommon for a muscle to be avulsed at its insertion as a result of pivoting, running, jumping, or twisting. Muscles that are frequently involved are the abdominals, hamstrings, and adductors of the leg (muscles that move the leg toward the midline of the body).

In individuals who have not completed growth, injuries to growth plates may occur with greater frequency than injuries to ligaments and bones. This is true because at this time in life, the growth plates are the weakest link in the musculoskeletal system. Such injuries frequently occur in athletics, where shearing forces are common.

The second type of fracture typically seen in skeletally immature individuals is an incomplete, or greenstick, fracture. In such fractures, the bone does not break completely due to its porous nature. The bone dissipates the force of the blow and may even bend without fracturing. Greenstick fractures do not usually occur in healthy, skeletally mature bone because it is strong and rigid and resists force.

Most fractures are the result of a direct force. Either an object strikes the person, or the person strikes the object, producing a fracture at the point of contact. Two additional causes are quite common in sport situations (see Figure 10.3). It is possible for indirect force to fracture a bone. The actual force may be applied to one part of the body (e.g., the hand) and be carried along bones to fracture another bone (e.g., the arm bone). This usually occurs in sports when the athlete uses his or her hand to "break" a fall. Twisting forces can also cause fractures. Football and skiing provide many examples of such injuries.

As noted in chapter 3, the cause, or mechanism, of injury is an important part of any injury assessment. You must consider the force of the impact, where it was applied, and the position of the athlete at impact. You, your assistant coaches, and the trainer should be especially watchful for twisting and hyperextension injuries, which often produce fractures that are undetected in the initial field assessment.

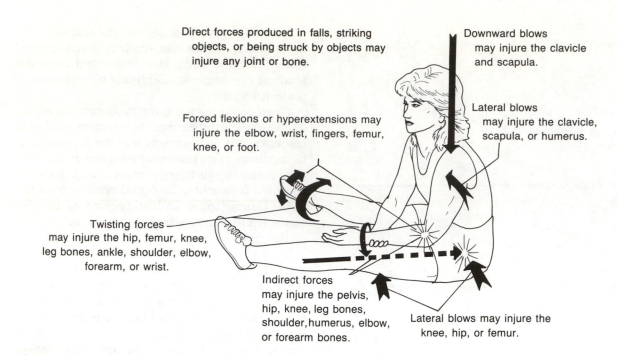

Direct forces produced in falls, striking objects, or being struck by objects may injure any joint or bone.

Downward blows may injure the clavicle and scapula.

Lateral blows may injure the clavicle, scapula, or humerus.

Forced flexions or hyperextensions may injure the elbow, wrist, fingers, femur, knee, or foot.

Twisting forces may injure the hip, femur, knee, leg bones, ankle, shoulder, elbow, forearm, or wrist.

Indirect forces may injure the pelvis, hip, knee, leg bones, shoulder, humerus, elbow, or forearm bones.

Lateral blows may injure the knee, hip, or femur.

Figure 10.3.   Mechanisms of injury for fractures.

Indications of a possible fracture include the following:

- *Sound of breaking.* The athlete or someone else has heard a sound (a "crack") indicating that a bone may have broken. When this happens, assume that there is a fracture.
- *Exposed bone.* An open fracture may show exposed bone ends or fragments.
- *Pain.* The athlete will complain of pain that is often severe at and adjacent to the injury site. Some fractures will produce very little pain at first, so do not assume that severe pain must be present.
- *Tenderness.* The area directly over the site will be very tender. Unless there is an open fracture or obvious deformity, you should use your fingertips gently to touch the area to determine tenderness and the exact location of the possible fracture.
- *Swelling.* Most fractures will produce some tissue swelling.
- *Discoloration.* The initial color change will be a reddening or a slight change in pigmentation. A black-and-blue bruise may not form until hours after the injury occurred. Typically the discoloration will drain toward the extremities (e.g., from the ankle to the toes), so you may see a larger area of discoloration as time goes on.

- *Deformity.* This may be obvious, especially when you compare the injured limb to the uninjured one. In some cases, you should gently feel along the area or the entire limb for lumps, bone fragments, or bone ends.
- *Loss of use.* The athlete may not be able to move a limb or a part of a limb, or the affected part can be moved but the movement produces intense pain. The athlete may guard the injured part to prevent movement. *Do not* ask the athlete to move the limb if you suspect a possible fracture as this may cause additional injury.
- *Tingling sensations or numbness.* These sensations may be the result of nerve or blood-vessel damage associated with a fracture.
- *Grating sounds or sensations.* You or the athlete may hear or feel grating when the injured limb is moved. *Do not* ask the athlete to move the injured limb to confirm grating.
- *Loss of distal pulse.* An artery may be severed or completely compressed by the pressure of bone ends or fragments. In addition to checking for pulse, you can check capillary refill by using the test described on page 56.

- *Loss of nerve function.* A nerve may be severed or may suffer a loss of function due to compression.
- *Muscle spasm.* Muscle spasms are the body's way of splinting an injured area to protect the involved tissue from further injury.

The damage to blood vessels and nerves is often more significant than the injury to the bone. For the upper extremities, determine if the injured arm has a radial pulse. If the injury involves the lower extremities, determine if a pulse can be felt behind the ankle bone on the inner side of the injured leg (posterior tibial pulse). Sometimes it is difficult to feel this pulse because of swelling. If accessible, check the nail beds using the capillary refill test. The absence of a distal pulse or taking longer than 2 seconds for capillary refill indicates either damage to major blood vessels or pressure being applied to these vessels.

Accurate determination of nerve function is very difficult under field conditions. Severe pain means possible nerve involvement. Do not ask the athlete to move, wave, lift, or push with the hand or foot of an injured limb. Simply touch a finger or toe on the injured limb and ask the athlete whether he or she can feel your touch and which digit was touched. You must assume that any negative answers are due to nerve damage (including the spinal cord) or pressure on the nerves.

WARNING:

If you suspect a fracture, dislocation, or crushing injury, do *not* remove the shoe. Touch an uninjured toe through the shoe.

Dislocations

A dislocation occurs whenever one end of a bone that makes up a joint is pulled out of place. The mechanism of injury is forceful, such as a blow or a twisting or pulling action. In some cases, the bone will also be fractured by the force that caused the dislocation. Soft tissues are damaged in *all* cases of dislocation. Recurrent dislocations are often caused by normal movements that would not have caused injury if the joint capsule were not stretched or torn. Because an adjoining bone may be fractured, treat all dislocations as seri-

ous injuries, including those that correct themselves.

A dislocation usually produces deformity at a joint with pain and swelling. In addition, muscle spasms cause excruciating pain and limit movement. Because of the extensive soft tissue damage, the accompanying muscle spasms, and the possibility of a fracture, always assume that there is a fracture when faced with these symptoms and signs, and provide the same care that you would for a fracture. Never attempt to realign a dislocation. Rather, splint the injured area as it lies.

Sprains and Strains

Ligaments are part of a joint's structure as they connect bone to bone. Whenever a ligament is partially torn, ruptured, or stretched, a sprain has occurred. *All* sprains that interfere with function should be considered to be serious. It is not possible to tell if the injury is a sprain, a fracture, a combination of the two, or if the young athlete has suffered a growth-plate injury in the field. Treat *all* moderate to severe sprains as if a fracture were present. The final determination must be made by a physician with X rays and other diagnostic techniques.

Strains were discussed in chapter 9. Since a strain occurs whenever a muscle is stretched, torn, or ruptured, this injury should be viewed as a soft-tissue injury. If the strain is severe, it must be treated in the same manner as a fracture.

It is often impossible to tell a severe strain from a sprain or fracture by using a simple field assessment. A sprain will typically produce swelling, some discoloration (often delayed up to 24 hours), and pain. In addition, there is usually pain on movement. Because these symptoms and signs mimic a fracture, you must treat all sprains that interfere with function as fractures. Similarly, the only sign of a strain often is pain and in many cases occurs only when the affected limb is moved. The safest approach is to treat all strains as possible fractures. Generally, most mild to moderate sport-related strains are obvious. Treat them as suggested in chapter 9. Severe strains must be treated as fractures because a stress fracture (see p. 106) or growth-plate injury may have occurred or the mechanism of injury may have produced a combined fracture and strain.

PROVIDING CARE

For all cases of possible fracture, dislocation, sprain, and severe strain, you must alert the EMS system. Most problems that require emergency care have a higher priority than do fractures. For example, an athlete who is unconscious and has a broken arm requires a different assessment and care than does one who is conscious and has suffered the same type of fracture. Make certain that you first assess the athlete for life-threatening problems. It is more important to detect respiratory and circulation problems, serious bleeding, developing shock, and possible neck and spinal injuries than it is to begin care immediately for a suspected fracture.

Preparation

Once the assessment indicates that the athlete's main problem is a probable skeletal injury, it is easy to want to immobilize (splint) the affected limb immediately. Instead of beginning by applying a splint, do the following:

1. Assign someone to alert the EMS system.
2. Reassure the athlete. Tell the athlete what you are doing, what you plan to do, and why these actions are necessary.
3. Safely control bleeding. Attempt to do this without placing pressure directly on the site of a possible fracture or dislocation. Expose the wound site if necessary.
4. Expose the injury site. Cut away or fold back clothing so that you can see the entire area of the affected part. Do *not* remove clothing by pulling it over an injured limb. Provide additional care, if needed, to control bleeding.
5. Remove jewelry from the injured limb.[1] Do *not* reposition the affected limb to remove jewelry as this can be done after splinting.
6. Dress and bandage any open wound at the injury site. Do not attempt to pick

bone fragments out of the wound or push bone ends back into an open wound.
7. Evaluate distal pulse and nerve function. Indications of severe blood-vessel or nerve damage may affect how you apply a splint.
8. Prepare all the materials needed to splint the injured limb. Continue with splinting procedures *only* if medical assistance will be delayed and you are trained in splinting techniques.
9. When splinting is required, *gently* reposition the limb. This is not done for all cases of possible fracture (see p. 119 and specific care in chapter 11). Remember that this is to be done only to allow for splint placement; otherwise, never move the injured limb.
10. Immobilize the affected part with a padded splint. To be effective, the splint should immobilize the injured bone and the joints above and below the bone. If a joint is injured, you must immobilize the joint and the bones above and below it.
11. Make certain that you splint firmly, securing the splint with a gauze roller bandage (start the wrap at the distal end of the limb). Do not apply the bandage too tightly as this will restrict circulation. Be sure to leave the tips of fingers or toes exposed to monitor skin-color and temperature changes that indicate restricted circulation.
12. Recheck distal pulse and nerve function.
13. Begin treating the athlete for shock even if there are no current indications of its development.
14. Continue to reassure the athlete.

Splinting

Splinting is a process that will immobilize a possible fracture or dislocation site, and a *splint* is used to provide this immobilization. There are two major types of splints:

- *Soft splints.* These are soft objects such as a sling or a pillow and can aid in immobilizing the injured part.
- *Rigid splints.* These are stiff objects that can be placed along an injured limb to

---

[1]An athlete should not be wearing jewelry during participation; however, some insist on doing so without the coach's knowledge. *Always* check the injured limb for jewelry.

stabilize the bone and the joints above and below it.

Splinting is an effort to reduce the complications associated with skeletal injury. Once in place, a splint can help keep bone ends from rubbing against, or placing pressure on, nerves and other sensitive tissues. This is seen in the fact that splinting often *reduces pain*. Splinting will help *reduce damage to soft tissues* by preventing movement of bone ends and restricting the movement of muscles and other soft tissues that may rub against bone ends or fragments. In fact, the process of immobilization can prevent closed fractures from becoming open ones.

Splinting is very important in protecting the circulation in the affected limb. It will *reduce the risk of bleeding* by helping to prevent damage to blood vessels, and it will *protect against restricted blood flow* by helping to prevent the compression of blood vessels by bone ends and fragments.

The splints that you use may be commercially manufactured splints, homemade splints, or items that are available on the scene. Figure 10.4 illustrates the many types of splints available. A wide variety of upper- and lower-extremity splint sets can be purchased. Rigid splints are most commonly used, but you also can buy commercial slings and inflatable splints.

Soft Splints

For certain types of upper-extremity injuries such as a fractured collarbone or dislocated shoulder, soft splinting is more practical than is rigid splinting. One variety of soft splint you can use is a sling and swathe. A sling is simply a triangular bandage that is large enough to support the arm. A swathe is a bandage that secures the arm and sling to the athlete's chest. You can use a commercial sling and swathe or make your own from cloth, toweling, a sheet, or clothing. To make a sling for an adult, the material should be folded or cut so that it forms a triangle that is 50-60 inches long at the base and 36-40 inches long on each side. The swathe must be long enough to be tied around the arm and chest.

Improvised splints

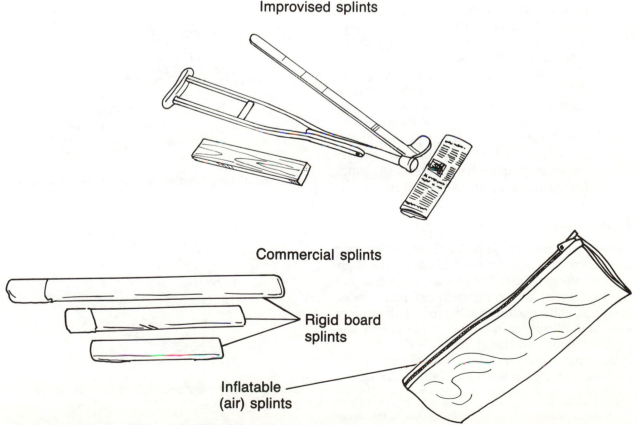

Commercial splints

Rigid board splints

Inflatable (air) splints

Figure 10.4. A variety of types of splints are available.

To apply a sling and swathe, follow the basic procedures for skeletal injury care and proceed in this manner:

1. Place the sling on the athlete's injured side and chest (see Figure 10.5). Leave enough material to the back so that the sling can extend beyond the elbow.

2. Set the athlete's arm across the chest and have him or her support the arm in this position.

3. Take the lower point of the triangle and pull it up over the athlete's arm to a position over the shoulder on the injured side.

4. Pull up on both ends of the sling so that the athlete's hand is about 4 inches above the elbow.[2]

5. Tie these two ends of the sling together so that the knot will rest over the neck or the top of the shoulder on the uninjured side. It is best to place a pad of dressing material or a handkerchief between the athlete and the knot. Be sure to leave the fingertips exposed. Check for a radial pulse and nerve function.

6. Create a pocket for the elbow by bringing forward the point that is behind the elbow and pinning it to the front of the sling. If you know that you do not have a pin, twist and knot this material before applying the sling.

7. Use a second piece of material, gauze roller bandage, Velcro straps, or other suitable item to create a swathe. The swathe should be about 4 inches wide. Tie the swathe so that it goes over the top of the injured limb and around the chest, staying to the outside of the sling. Leave the uninjured limb free.

Rigid Splints

These splints *must* be padded before they are applied to the injured limb. Some have their own washable pads. If necessary, you can pad rigid splints by wrapping them in a gauze roller bandage. The padding will protect the injury site and allow for a better fit between the injured limb and the splint.

You can make your own rigid splints or improvise a splint if none is available at an injury

---

[2]This angle varies depending on the nature of the injury (see chapter 11 for specifics).

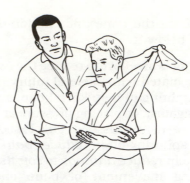

1
Place sling on chest and fold injured limb across.

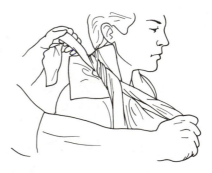

2
Draw up ends, raising athlete's hand 4 inches above elbow.

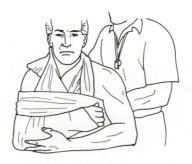

3
Tie ends of sling together over top of pad.

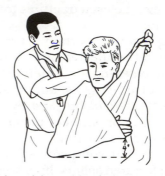

4
Swathe around chest and injured limb. Keep the uninjured limb free.

Figure 10.5.   Applying a sling and swathe.

scene. Splints can be made from plywood or other lumber products, cardboard, rolled newspapers or magazines, and tongue depressors (for fractured fingers). In the past, people have improvised splints from shin guards, hockey sticks, canes, umbrellas, brooms, and shovel handles. The item used must be stiff enough to give support to the injured limb and long enough to immobilize the bone and the joint above and below it (or the joint and the bones above and below it). Many homemade and improvised splints are inadequate because they are too short.

Follow the basic procedures for skeletal injury care. When you place the splint along the injured limb, *gently* reposition the limb to apply the splint.

Do *not* attempt to reposition the limb for splinting if

- there is obvious angulation;
- the injury involves the shoulder, elbow, wrist, hand, pelvis, hip, knee, ankle, or foot (see chapter 11);
- the repositioning causes additional severe pain; or
- the limb resists your first attempt.

Do not attempt to reposition a fractured thigh or a lower leg if there is either an angulated or an open thigh fracture.

In these instances, splint the injured area as you found it. Do not attempt to realign joints or limb segments.

Inflatable Splints

These splints may be used to immobilize possible fractures of the forearm and lower leg. Inflatable splints are easy to use but do present a number of serious problems. You must be certain that they will be able to hold air before they are used. Some inflatable splints tend to develop leaks as they age. In addition, the splints may be accidentally damaged in storage. Sometimes these problems are not noticed until the splint is in place. The pressure in the splint must be monitored in the event there is a leak. Also, inflatable splints may not be returned to you because they have to be cut off the athlete once care begins at a medical facility.

To apply an inflatable splint, you should follow the basic procedures for skeletal injury care and take these steps:

1. Start with an *uninflated* splint that you have slipped over your forearm (see Figure 10.6).
2. Have someone support the injured limb while you *gently* straighten it to allow application of the splint (follow the restrictions listed previously).
3. Slide the splint off your forearm and directly onto the athlete's injured limb.

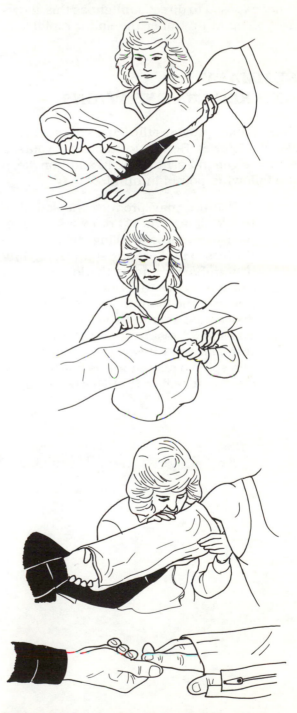

Figure 10.6. Applying an inflatable splint.

4. Smooth out the splint so that there are no wrinkles and inflate it by mouth or by using the pump supplied by the manufacturer. The splint is properly inflated when you can make a small surface indentation with your finger.

Keep monitoring the pressure in the splint, check for nerve and circulatory function, and make certain that the athlete's splinted limb is not exposed to direct sunlight as this allows heat to build up under the splint rapidly.

SUMMARY AND RECOMMENDATIONS

This chapter provides the basics in the care of skeletal injuries. Be sure to familiarize yourself with the general principles. In addition, keep the following points in mind:

1. A fracture may produce the sound of breaking (a "crack") or exposed bone, pain, tenderness, swelling, discoloration, the loss of use, grating sounds, tingling or numbness, and/or the loss of distal pulse or nerve function.
2. Because the symptoms and signs of a dislocation mimic those of a fracture, you should assume that there is a fracture and treat it accordingly. Remember, splint a dislocation as it lies. Do not attempt to realign it. *All* dislocations are serious injuries even if the dislocation corrects itself. Similarly, treat all moderate to severe sprains and serious strains as if there were a fracture.
3. Alert the EMS system for all cases of possible fracture, dislocation, sprain that interferes with function, and serious strain. Do the necessary assessment and care for life-threatening emergencies, bleeding, developing shock, possible spinal injury, and open wounds before immobilizing possible fractures.
4. Proper wound care will require that you cut or lift away clothing that is over the injury site to allow a clear view of the affected area.
5. Distal pulse and nerve-action assessments must be made before and after splinting.
6. Always treat the athlete for the development of shock even if there are no indications of it occurring.
7. Splints are used to immobilize the injured bone and the joints above and below it (or the injured joint and the bones above and below it). You can select among soft (e.g., sling and swathe), rigid, and inflatable splints. Make certain that the splints you use are long enough and that all rigid splints are padded. Inflatable splints must be monitored to ensure that the correct amount of pressure is being applied.

Chapter 11
Skeletal Injury Care—The Extremities

When an EMS or other health care professional response is available within 10 minutes, you should not splint an injured extremity as this may prevent the medical staff from making a full assessment or may delay transport if your splint must be removed and another splint applied. Check with your local EMS system to determine the estimated response time to reach the places where you will be practicing and competing. Follow their guidelines as to when you should splint or when you should wait.

In the situation in which you will not be splinting, remember to assess the injuries, care for life-threatening emergencies, protect the neck and spine (when appropriate), control bleeding, care for open wounds, and treat for developing shock. Reassure the athlete and protect him or her from additional injury. You should *not* move the unsplinted athlete who may have skeletal injuries. If there are no indications of neck or spinal injury, the splinted, stable athlete can be moved (see chapters 12 and 15).

Remember to assess distal pulse and nerve function before and after splinting. If there is a loss of pulse or nerve function after a splint is applied, you will have to loosen and reapply the ties that secure the splint to see whether pulse or function is restored. If this does not restore the pulse or nerve function, resplinting will be necessary.

If there is no pulse or nerve function when you assess the athlete's injured limb, you should wait for medical assistance to arrive. If splinting is necessary, it may restore the pulse or function.

More advanced training than that provided in this book can teach you how to use manual traction (tension) placed along the long axis of the affected limb to restore pulse or nerve function in cases that do not involve the ankle or wrist. Such training is usually a part of EMS training programs and should not be tried without the benefit of training.

THE UPPER EXTREMITIES

The basic principles of assessment and splinting described in chapter 10 apply to the care of the upper extremities. If you will be splinting the injured athlete, remember that joint injuries require a cautious, gentle approach.

The Shoulder Girdle

When assessing injuries to the shoulder girdle, check for the general signs of fracture and dislocation at the collarbone (clavicle), shoulder blade (scapula), humerus, shoulder joint, tip of the shoulder, breastbone (sternum), and the joint formed by the collarbone and breastbone. Fractures specific to the shoulder girdle are fractures to the collarbone and the shoulder blade.

The fractured collarbone is the most common fracture in children and is produced by the direct force of straight-on impact, an impact from above, or an indirect force applied to the shoulder during a fall. The fractured shoulder blade is rare and is usually caused by a direct blow over the top of the bone or a downward blow to the shoulder.

In addition to the typical symptoms and signs of skeletal injuries, examine the athlete for the following conditions:

- Deformity along the collarbone (clavicle) or where the collarbone attaches to the breastbone (sternum) and shoulder blade (scapula). (This will help you to assess possible fractures and dislocations.) Pay particular attention to the medial end of the collarbone next to the breastbone. It is the last growth area to close, closing between the ages of 23 and 35. A posterior dislocation of the joint formed by the breastbone and collarbone (sternoclavicular joint) could be life threatening because the esophagus, the trachea, and major blood vessels and nerves lie directly behind the joint. Sports are the second most common cause of dislocations in this joint.
- "Dropped" shoulder, in which the injured shoulder will appear to be knocked downward while the athlete holds the arm against the chest. (This indicates a possible fracture to the collarbone, a dislocated shoulder, or a sprain of the joint at the lateral end of the collarbone, or the acromioclavicular joint.) In moderate to severe sprains of the acromioclavicular joint you will see a bump at the tip of the shoulder. This is the lateral end of the collarbone, which is no longer held tightly in place because some of the restraining ligaments have been torn.
- Loss of the rounded contour of the shoulder and a bulge that can be seen on the chest wall just below the collarbone. (The bulge is the upper end of the arm bone, or humerus. Its position indicates an anterior inferior dislocation of the shoulder.)
- Pain and tenderness over the shoulder blade. (Do not lift an injured athlete who is supine to make this examination.) If the athlete complains of pain and tenderness following a blow to the upper back, assume a possible fracture and immobilize the limb on the affected side using a sling and swathe.

Carry out the basic assessment and care procedures for the injury and, when it is your responsibility, splint. Remember to check for circulatory and nerve function before and after splinting. If soft splinting is to be done, apply a sling and swathe (p. 118). If there are any indications of an anterior dislocation, place a pillow, a pad of rolled towel, or a blanket between the injured arm and the chest before placing and securing the sling. Rigid splinting is not practical for shoulder girdle injuries.

WARNING:

A dislocated shoulder may correct (reduce) itself. If this happens, follow the basic care procedures for an injured shoulder girdle, then splint. You must request an EMS response. There may be severe tissue damage even if there are no symptoms or signs of serious injury. Do *not* attempt to straighten dislocations or angulations of the shoulder. Do not try to "pop" the shoulder back into place. To do so may cause severe damage to major blood vessels and nerves that pass near the joint.

The Upper Arm

The most common mechanism of injury to the arm is an indirect force carried by the hand and arm when the athlete falls and strikes the ground or floor with the hand. Direct force to the arm also will produce fractures. The child athlete often suffers a dislocation, while the adolescent or young adult may have a dislocation complicated by fractures. The adult athlete usually suffers a fracture.

Deformity and tenderness are key signs in detecting a possible fracture of the upper-arm bone (humerus). Perform the necessary assessment and follow the general procedures for skeletal injury care. Be alert to the possibility of epiphyseal separations at both the proximal (upper) and distal (lower) ends of the humerus. The proximal epiphysis closes between the ages of 18 and 21 and the distal epiphysis between 14 and 18.

Rigid Splinting

The best method of care for a skeletal injury of the upper arm bone is to apply a rigid splint

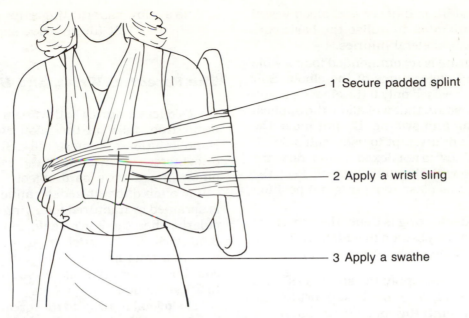

1 Secure padded splint

2 Apply a wrist sling

3 Apply a swathe

Figure 11.1. Techniques for splinting a fracture of the humerus: rigid splinting with a sling and swathe.

along with a sling and modified swathe (see Figure 11.1). Use a splint that will extend from above the shoulder to a point below the elbow. Have someone steady the injured limb above and below the injury site while you place the padded splint along the lateral surface of the arm. Secure the splint to the injured arm beginning at the distal end of the splint. You may use a gauze roller bandage, cloth ties (cravats), or handkerchiefs.

Place a roll of dressing or cloth in the palm of the injured limb to maintain the hand's *position of function*, which is the position that the palm and fingers would assume when trying to grasp a small ball. Reassess distal pulse and nerve function. If these have been lost, you will have to resplint.

After rigid splinting, place a pad or a small pillow between the injured arm and chest and apply a sling and narrow swathe. Reassess distal pulse and nerve function.

Soft Splinting

Soft splinting requires applying a sling and swathe. The method of application to use depends on the injury site. When the injury is near the shoulder, apply a standard sling and swathe. For injuries along the shaft, apply a wrist sling and swathe (see Figure 11.2). Do not draw the hand upward. If the injury is near the elbow, treat as a fractured elbow.

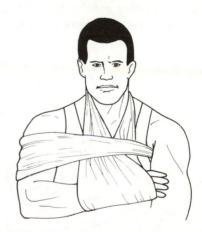

Figure 11.2. The wrist sling and swathe.

The Elbow

Most elbow fractures are caused by a fall on an outstretched hand, as are dislocations of the joint. Dislocations, however, can also result from a severe direct blow. Major nerves and blood vessels, which pass close to the upper-arm bone (humerus) across the front of the elbow, are susceptible to damage both in fractures involving the humerus and in elbow dislocations. Be sure to check nerve and circulatory function in all injuries involving the elbow during your assessment and before and after splinting.

The elbow *must* be splinted in the position in which it is found as any changes in position may cause additional nerve and blood vessel damage. Remember to utilize the basic care procedures for skeletal injuries.

Rigid splinting is recommended for possible fractures and dislocations of the elbow. Soft splinting can be used only if the elbow is found in a flexed position that will allow the application of a sling and swathe. Do *not* move the athlete's arm or attempt to use a soft splint if the injured elbow is not flexed. Do not raise the hand upward with the sling. Instead, keep the elbow flexion as close to its original position as possible.

When rigid splinting is done, the arm must be splinted in the position in which it is found. Two options follow (see Figure 11.3):

- *Elbow flexed.* Apply the splint as shown in Figure 11.3a. Provide support for the splinted limb by placing a pillow or blanket under the upper arm.
- *Arm straight or not properly flexed for other splinting methods.* Secure a padded splint that extends from the armpit

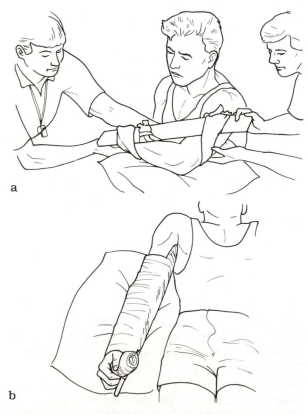

a

b

Figure 11.3. Splints used for stabilizing elbow fractures: (a) rigid board splint with upper arm flexed at the elbow; (b) long splint used with the arm straight.

to a point past the fingertips as shown in Figure 11.3b (do not use a shorter splint).

The Forearm, Wrist, and Hand

Most skeletal injuries to the forearm and wrist occur from falls on the outstretched hand. Hand injuries are most often the result of direct forces, such as the hand being stepped on or hit against a hard object.

It is often difficult to determine if the wrist is sprained or fractured following a fall, particularly when there is no deformity. If there is tenderness in the wrist, treat the injury as if it were a fracture. Injury to the growth area could be present in athletes younger than 17 to 19 years of age.

For skeletal injuries to the forearm, wrist, or hand, apply the basic procedures for skeletal injury care and splint.

WARNING:

Do *not* attempt to straighten the injured wrist or hand.

When possible, use rigid splints. However, if soft splinting must be done, fold a pillow or a blanket around the athlete's injured forearm, wrist, and hand and apply a standard sling and swathe or tie the forearm and hand between two pillows. Although rigid splinting is preferable, soft splinting may be done for fractures to the elbow end of the forearm or for those to the wrist and hand. Injuries along the shafts of the forearm bones or at the wrist end of the forearm need rigid splinting.

A padded rigid splint can be applied to immobilize the forearm, wrist, and hand, and it must extend from beyond the elbow to a point past the fingertips (see Figure 11.4). A roll of dressing or cloth should be used to keep the hand in the position of function. A sling and swathe can be added to provide additional support and protection for the splinted limb.

The Fingers

Injuries to the fingers usually are caused by forced flexion or extension, direct blows, or

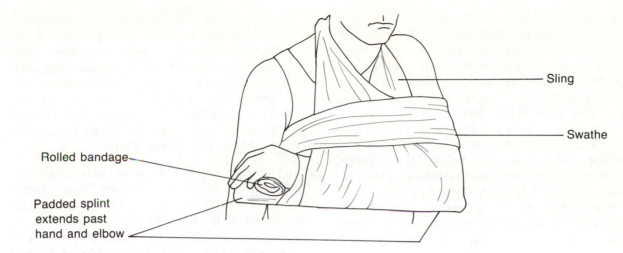

Sling

Swathe

Rolled bandage

Padded splint
extends past
hand and elbow

Figure 11.4. Rigid splinting of the forearm.

crushing forces. If there is no damage to the rest of the extremity and the injury is to the most extreme end of the finger, simply tape the injured finger to an adjacent uninjured finger. A tongue depressor can be used as a splint for an injured finger (see Figure 11.5) and can be secured to the finger using a gauze roller bandage, cloth ties, or tape. If the injury is to the middle segment of the finger or closer to the hand, splint the finger in a flexed position over a rolled bandage. Regardless of the method used to immobilize the finger, additional protection should be offered by placing the affected limb in a sling and swathe.

WARNING:

Do *not* try to treat dislocated fingers by "popping" them back into their sockets but provide the same care that you would for a fracture. Such dislocations are sometimes associated with a chip fracture, which could result in a bone chip becoming caught in the joint during the attempt to reduce the dislocation. The dislocation could also be an epiphyseal separation. These epiphyses close between the ages of 14 and 21.

"Buddy taping," taping the injured finger to an adjacent uninjured finger, is an easy way of protecting the injured finger when the athlete returns to activity. Try to keep the index finger free to avoid injury and allow for maximized performance.

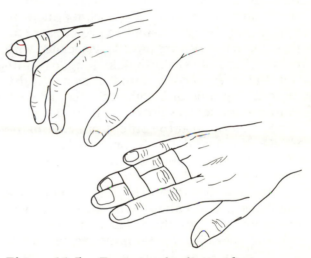

Figure 11.5. Taping and splinting finger injuries.

THE LOWER EXTREMITIES

The basic principles of skeletal injury care apply to the lower extremities. In addition to the standard cautions concerning joints, the coach must be aware of the gentle handling required to care for pelvic injuries. Keep in mind that any injury that fractures the pelvis, dislocates the hip, or fractures the thigh bone is usually severe enough to have caused some kind of spinal damage. In addition, always treat the individual for shock.

The Pelvic Girdle

The major skeletal injuries to the pelvic girdle involve pelvic fractures, hip fractures (the head of the femur and/or the joint surface of the pelvis), and hip dislocations. Sport-related pelvic fractures are rare; however, the force produced by falls from apparatus (including straddling falls) or by diving can fracture pelvic bones. Pelvic fractures are slow to heal and often meet with complications.

Most serious pelvic fractures are related to falls. Remember that falls on the buttocks may produce pelvic fractures. Any fall that renders the athlete unconscious must be considered to have produced enough force to fracture the pelvis and/or cause spinal injuries. Direct blows to the pelvis and to the outside of the thigh (lateral) or the hip also may produce fractures or dislocations.

Avulsion fractures (see p. 91) can occur at the pelvis. These are seen most frequently in the child and the young adolescent athlete, in which case they are usually a growth area injury. Such injuries are usually associated with running (mainly sprinting), kicking, or jumping that stretches the hamstrings or quadriceps. Symptoms and signs may be delayed. Pain and tenderness are typically present and are often located at the outer front edge of the pelvis, at or near the groin, or at the lower edge of the buttocks. The athlete must be examined by a physician.

Direct blows to the hip or thigh can produce fractures or dislocations. The dislocation will often produce a fracture. The symptoms and signs of possible skeletal injury to the pelvic girdle include the following:

- Pain in the pelvis, hip, and/or thigh
- Pain when pressure is applied to the wings of the pelvis (Apply this pressure gently by placing your hands on the lateral wings, or the upper sides, of the pelvis. Warn the athlete that there may be some pain as you lightly compress the wings and note any painful response or any area of deformity. Do not apply this pressure if there is obvious injury or other indications of pelvic girdle injury.)
- Deformity of the pelvis (rare) or the hip joint
- The athlete reports that he or she cannot lift the leg while lying on the back (Do not ask the athlete to attempt to demonstrate this fact.)
- The foot on the injured side is turned outward
- The entire leg is rotated outward (This

often is an indication of an anterior hip dislocation, but may also indicate a hip fracture. In some cases, the injured limb may appear to be shorter than the limb on the uninjured side. When this is observed, you must suspect a hip fracture.)
- The entire limb is rotated inward and the knee is bent (This indicates a possible posterior hip dislocation.)

If there are any indications of pelvic fracture, hip fracture, or hip dislocation, do not move the athlete and do not lift or reposition the lower limbs. Severe blood-vessel, nerve, and perhaps internal organ damage may occur with movement. Remember that any force that is powerful enough to injure the pelvis or hip severely also may have produced spinal and/or internal injuries. Always treat for shock, but do *not* move the athlete or elevate the lower extremities.

In most cases that involve pelvic girdle fractures or dislocations, keep the athlete protected and at rest and wait for medical assistance to arrive. Some protection from movement can be offered if you carefully place rolled blankets, pillows, rolled towels, or folded clothing along the sides of the lower extremities without moving the athlete.

The Thigh

The most common cause of thigh fractures is a direct blow to the thigh or the knee. Many of these fractures are open fractures that will require you to control bleeding and provide open-wound care. You should carry out these steps even if you do not plan to splint. Closed-thigh fractures may have profuse internal bleeding. Whenever there is a possible thigh fracture, open or closed, treat for shock but do not lift the lower limbs. Remember that a force that is strong enough to damage the thigh bone also may have caused pelvic and spinal injuries.

There is no soft-splinting procedure for skeletal injuries of the thigh, and, while rigid splinting can be done, in most cases it is best to wait for medical assistance to arrive. Trained personnel will apply a special splint called a traction splint, which is designed to provide the care needed for thigh fractures. If a traction splint is available, do not attempt to use it as they are meant to be used only by trained emergency care professionals. If an EMS response will be delayed, you can apply a rigid splint, but be very careful. Make no attempt to splint if there are any indications of spinal, pelvic, or hip involvement. Such complications are possible in most cases.

Thigh splinting requires the entire lower limb to be immobilized. Use one long, well-padded splint that extends from the athlete's armpit to a point beyond the foot. Additional padding should be placed in the armpit prior to applying the splint. Do not move the athlete or the lower limbs to place the ties for securing the splint. Instead, slide the ties under the void at the waist and the knee using a flat splint or coat hanger and carefully slide them into the tying positions. Do not place a tie over any possible fracture site. A more effective way to immobilize is to use a second, rigid splint (see Figure 11.6). This splint must be long enough to extend from the crotch to a point beyond the foot. Before it is set in place, additional padding must be placed in the groin area.

The Knee

Direct blows to the knee from any side, direct blows from a fall, twisting forces (or forced rotation), and indirect forces applied usually by landing on the feet can cause skeletal injury to the knee. Hyperextension, and sometimes hyperflexion, can also produce skeletal injuries to the knee. If the kneecap (patella) is fractured, this is usually the result of a fall onto the knee. Serious trauma to the thigh may produce severe muscle contractions that may cause additional injury.

Field assessments cannot determine if a knee injury is a sprain, an epiphyseal separation (growth injury), a fracture, or a dislocation. Prior to the age of 16 to 19, the epiphysis of the lower end of the femur (thighbone) is open and susceptible to injury from a blow to the outside of the knee. Do *not* reposition or attempt to straighten the lower limb during your assessment or splinting. Splint the knee in the position in which it is found. Soft splinting is not recommended for knee injuries. Make sure you check for nerve and circulatory function immediately. Many nerves and major blood vessels pass close to the knee joint.

When rigid splinting is done, the basic principles of skeletal injury care must be followed. During the splinting procedures, make certain that someone is stabilizing the injured limb. Make every effort to reduce leg movement.

If the knee is bent, place a padded splint along the outside (lateral) surface of the limb. Secure it in place at the thigh and lower leg. The splinted limb can be rested on a pillow or folded blankets (see Figure 11.7). More effective splinting can be done if two splints are applied to care for the knee injury. One should be placed on the outer surface and one on the inner surface of the limb. These splints should be secured at the same time.

If the knee is straight, apply a padded rigid splint that is long enough to extend from the armpit to a point beyond the foot. In an emergency, a shorter splint may be used, but it *must* extend from the athlete's waist to beyond the foot. Make certain that you pad the armpit before placing the splint. Use cloth ties to secure the splint at the chest, waist, thigh, above the knee, below the knee, at midcalf and at the ankle (see Figure 11.8).

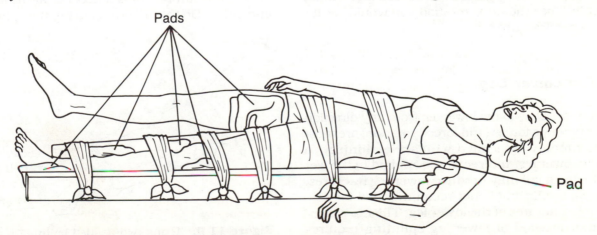

Figure 11.6. Using two rigid splints to stabilize a fractured femur.

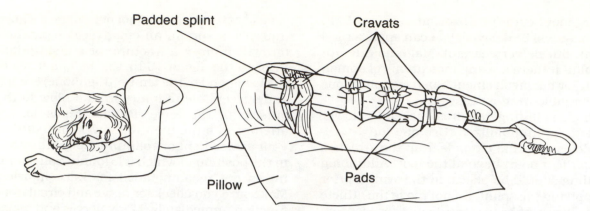

Figure 11.7. Splinting an injured knee with the knee flexed.

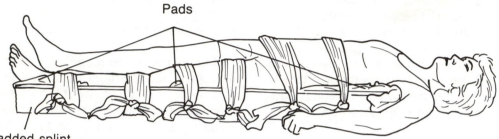

Figure 11.8. Splinting an injured knee with the leg straight.

A dislocated kneecap (patella) is often considered to be a minor injury. But even when the dislocation corrects itself (the kneecap pops back into place), an EMS response is necessary, and the athlete *must* be examined by a physician. Frequently, once the patella dislocates, it can become recurrent and still requires medical attention. In addition, there could be serious injuries that may not be apparent for hours or even days. Unless there will be a long delay in the EMS response, do not splint. Keep the athlete at rest. If you must splint, use the same method you would use for a knee fracture.

the outside (lateral) and one on the inside (medial) surface of the leg (see Figure 11.9). This can be difficult to manage. The splinting process is best done if you have someone stabilize the athlete's lower limb and someone else hold the splints. The splints must be padded and must be long enough to extend from above the knee to below the foot. Secure both splints in place at the same time using cloth strips or a gauze roller bandage. The splints will be more effective if you place gauze or cloth padding in the natural voids that occur at the knee and ankle. Do this before securing the splints.

The Lower Leg

A direct blow to the lower leg from any direction or twisting forces (and forced rotation) are most commonly associated with skeletal injury to the lower leg. Indirect force applied to the feet during a fall may produce lower leg fractures.

Soft splinting is not recommended for possible fractures of the lower leg. The most common method of lower-leg splinting requires placing two padded rigid splints with one on

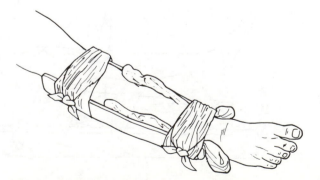

Figure 11.9. Using two padded splints to stabilize the lower leg.

The Ankle and Foot

The weight borne by the ankle and the forces applied to this joint during sports activities make it very susceptible to skeletal injury. Direct blows, twisting forces, and indirect blows (usually from falls) can produce such an injury. In addition, growth area injuries are common because the distal epiphyses of the tibia and fibula remain open until between the ages of 17 and 18.

The foot can suffer skeletal injury as a result of direct blows, twisting forces, or stress placed on the foot when it is flexed, extended, or rotated. The heel bone (calcaneus) and toes (metatarsals) are the most commonly fractured bones in sport-related ankle and foot injuries. Many of these fractures are stress fractures resulting from jumping, walking, or running. Fractures involving the heel are frequently caused by falls where the athlete lands on the heel. Severe hyperextensions or flexions of the foot may also produce skeletal injury. Always splint the ankle in the position in which it is found.

For most cases, soft splinting is the best method for immobilizing an injured ankle or foot. Wrap a pillow around the ankle and foot and tie this in place with strips of cloth, a gauze roller bandage, or pieces of clothing (as shown in Figure 11.10). If a pillow is not available, use folded blankets that are of the same

thickness as a pillow. If rigid splinting is done, use the same method employed for a fracture of the lower leg provided the ankle is in alignment with the lower leg.

SUMMARY AND RECOMMENDATIONS

Splinting by coaches is usually done only when there is a long wait for an EMS response. The athlete cannot be moved until splinting is completed.

In addition to the standard symptoms and signs associated with skeletal injuries, there are some special signs of injury to the shoulder girdle and the pelvic girdle:

Shoulder Girdle

- Deformity along the collarbone (possible fracture or dislocation)
- Pain and tenderness over the top of the shoulder blade (possible fracture)
- "Dropped" shoulder (possible clavicular fracture, shoulder dislocation, or dislocation of the collarbone)
- Deformity or movement caused by the top of the arm bone (possible anterior inferior dislocation)

Pelvic Girdle

- Pain when the wings of the pelvis are compressed (possible pelvic fracture)
- Inability to lift the leg while on the back (possible fracture or dislocation; do not request that the athlete demonstrate this failure)
- Foot rotated outward associated with pelvic or hip injury (possible pelvic fracture)
- Limb rotated outward (possible anterior hip dislocation or hip fracture)
- Limb rotated inward with knee bent (possible posterior hip dislocation)

Skeletal injury care is reviewed in Figure 11.11 on page 130.

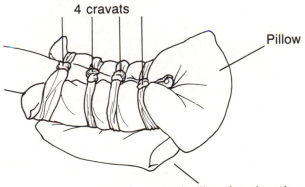

4 cravats

Pillow

2nd pillow for elevation

Figure 11.10.   The pillow splint.

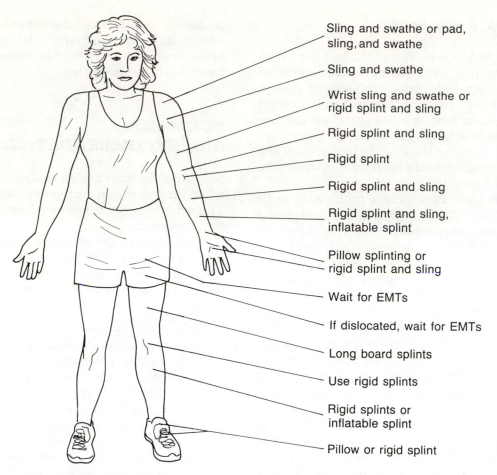

Sling and swathe or pad, sling, and swathe

Sling and swathe

Wrist sling and swathe or rigid splint and sling

Rigid splint and sling

Rigid splint

Rigid splint and sling

Rigid splint and sling, inflatable splint

Pillow splinting or rigid splint and sling

Wait for EMTs

If dislocated, wait for EMTs

Long board splints

Use rigid splints

Rigid splints or inflatable splint

Pillow or rigid splint

Figure 11.11. Review of skeletal injury care.

Chapter 12
Skeletal Injury Care—The Skull, Spine, and Chest

Injuries to the head, spine, or chest may render the athlete unconscious. In these cases, assume that a spinal injury has occurred. Do not move or reposition the athlete unless it is necessary for providing basic life support. Protect the unconscious athlete from the elements, including direct sunlight. If the eyes of the unconscious athlete are open and are not injured, close them by exerting light pressure on the eyelids. If there is eye injury that prevents this action, the eyes will have to be covered.

Do not use ammonia caps in an attempt to arouse the unconscious athlete as this may cause the athlete to jerk his or her head and cause additional injury to the head, neck, or spine.

THE SKULL

The axial skeleton (see Figure 12.1) is made up of the skull, spine, ribs, and breastbone. The skull consists of the cranium, which holds and protects the brain, and the face. There are no moveable joints between cranial bones. The bones of the face form part of the eye sockets, the upper bony part of the nose, the cheeks, and the upper and lower jaws. The bone of the lower jaw (mandible) is the only moveable bone of the face.

Most head injuries that are sport-related involve the soft tissues only, making injuries that require an EMS response rare. Keep in mind that any history of head injury makes a new head injury potentially more dangerous.

Skeletal injuries of the skull include cranial fractures, facial fractures, and dislocations of the mandible and must always be considered serious since they may include airway obstruction and brain or spinal injury. Great care must be taken in caring for these injuries as they often heal slowly and infection could turn a minor injury into a life-threatening one.

Cranial Injuries

The danger of brain damage associated with head trauma makes any head injury potentially serious. The brain may be injured directly or indirectly. A *direct brain injury* occurs when the cranium is fractured and the brain is

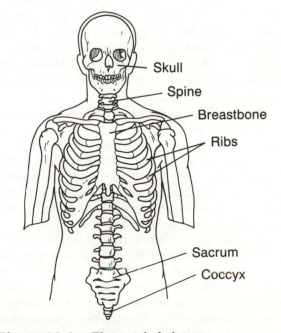

Figure 12.1. The axial skeleton.

damaged by pieces of bone or a foreign object. This can happen with the scalp remaining intact. *Indirect brain injury* occurs when the cranium remains intact but the force is transmitted through the skull to the brain. Cranial injuries can be caused by a blow to the chin or head or a severe fall on the buttocks.

Types of Indirect Brain Injury

There are two major types of indirect brain injury—concussions and bruising (contusions). A *concussion* is a closed head injury that usually causes minor damage to the brain. Concussions are common injuries in contact sports, and their consequences are not easily detectable. In most cases, the athlete will feel groggy immediately after a blow to the head. A headache may develop, and there may or may not be a short-term loss of consciousness. Typically, unconsciousness will not recur. In some cases, there may be a temporary short-term memory loss that causes the athlete to be unaware of recent events (including the accident that produced the head injury). Temporary long-term memory loss is rare.

Fully assess the athlete for any indications of cranial or brain damage as listed in the next two sections. Make certain that you ask the athlete about recent and past events (e.g., "What is your name?" "Who are we playing?" "What is the score?" "How old are you?" "What day of the week is this?" and so on).

The symptoms and signs of a concussion may develop quickly or take hours or days to become obvious. Regardless of when the symptoms and signs appear, the athlete should receive EMS or other professional evaluation and should be transported to a medical facility if necessary.

A bruised brain, or *contusion*, occurs as part of a closed head injury when force is transmitted to the brain and ruptures blood vessels on the surface of the brain or deep within it. Because there is little free space inside the cranial cavity, an impact applied to one side of the head may force the brain into the bones on the opposite side, thus bruising the brain.

The symptoms and signs of a bruised brain are often severe and include prolonged unconsciousness or repeated lapses into unconsciousness. In some cases, the signs may be slow to develop or may mimic a concussion. Any indication of a bruised brain means that the athlete will require EMS transport to a medical facility.

Symptoms and Signs of Cranial Injury

A fractured skull may or may not be obvious. The mechanism of injury should be considered along with certain symptoms and signs that you can detect using the survey methods presented in chapter 3. You must assume that the athlete has a serious head injury if the blow to the head produces any of the following:

- A decreased level of awareness
- Unconsciousness (even if temporary)
- A large bruise or deep cut on the scalp or forehead
- Severe pain or swelling at the injury site
- Depressions, large swellings, or a deformed shape of the cranium
- A bruise behind the ear (may appear minor but is a serious sign)
- Discoloration under the eyes
- One or both eyes sunken
- Pupils unequally dilated and/or unresponsive to light
- Bleeding from the ears or bleeding from the nose that appears to be more than a simple nosebleed
- Clear or bloody fluids running from the ears and/or nose (may be the fluid that surrounds the brain, thus signifying a skull fracture)
- Progressive deterioration of pulse and breathing

Symptoms and Signs of Brain Injury

An injury to the head may have produced brain damage if you note any of the following conditions:

- Any sign of a cranial fracture
- Loss of consciousness, altered states of awareness, or personality changes
- A pulse that changes from slow and full to fast and weak
- Changes in the pattern of breathing (usually breathing that becomes rapid and then stops for a few seconds)
- Unequally dilated or unresponsive pupils
- Impaired vision, hearing, or sense of balance
- Loss of sensation or paralysis (might occur on one side of the body or be limited to one part of the body)
- Difficulties with speech
- Headache
- Forceful (projectile) vomiting

Cranial Injury Care

Any severe blow to the head that may have produced a cranial injury can also produce a spinal injury. If the athlete is unconscious or there are indications of a skull fracture or brain injury, assume that spinal injuries exist. *Do not* move or reposition an athlete who may have a serious skull or brain injury unless you must do so to provide basic cardiac life support. If the athlete has a minor head injury with no possibility of spinal involvement, he or she should be placed on the side with the head turned to allow drainage from the mouth and nose (see Figure 12.2). Do not place the athlete on the back or on the back with the upper body elevated as this could cause serious problems should the athlete vomit. Remember that vomiting often occurs following a head injury.

When providing care for an athlete with possible cranial fractures or brain injury, you should make certain that someone alerts the EMS system, reassure the athlete throughout care, and take the following steps:

1. Maintain an open airway using the jaw-thrust procedure when necessary (see p. 38). Stay alert for vomiting.
2. Provide rescue breathing or CPR if necessary. Injury to the brain may cause a quick onset of breathing and heart failure.
3. Keep the athlete at rest and do not allow the athlete to reposition him- or herself.
4. Control bleeding using direct pressure and a dressing. Do *not* apply pressure over the injury site if there are bone fragments, depressions, or exposed brain tissue at the site. Instead, loosely apply a bulky dressing.

5. Stabilize any penetrating objects.
6. Dress any open wounds. Do *not* remove bone fragments or debris from the wound site.
7. Treat for shock but do not lift the legs. Remember, there may be spinal injuries.
8. Continue to monitor pulse and breathing and note any changes in the athlete's level of awareness. Changes of pulse rate and character, breathing rate and character, and level of awareness are very significant and must be reported to the medical professionals.

WARNING:

Do *not* try to stop the flow of clear or bloody fluids from the nose or the flow of blood, bloody fluids, or clear fluids from the ear. Place a sterile, loose dressing at the ear opening or the nostrils to help prevent additional contamination.

WARNING:

Emergency care professionals now consider the removal of a helmet from the head of an athlete who may have serious head or spinal injuries to be a specialized skill. In most cases, you will be able to remove a face mask and ensure an adequate airway and provide basic care. Do *not* remove the helmet of any unconscious athlete or one who may have suffered a possible head or spinal injury.

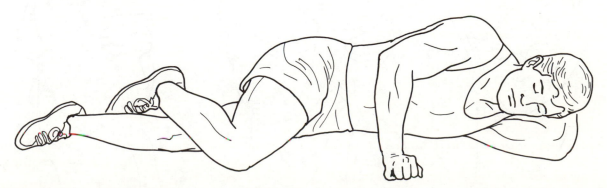

Figure 12.2. If the athlete has no possibility of spinal injury, you can position him or her on the side to allow adequate drainage.

Facial Injuries

Most facial injuries are soft-tissue injuries; however, facial fractures and lower-jaw dislocations do occur in sports. A severe blow, such as that produced in a fall from apparatus or the striking of the side of the pool during a dive, is usually required to produce these injuries. These injuries also have been associated with being struck in the face by a hard ball, bat, or stick. Loose and avulsed teeth are discussed in chapter 7. Eye injuries are covered in chapter 7.

Symptoms and Signs of Facial Bone Injury

Any severe blow to the face may cause facial fractures and be transmitted to produce spinal injury. A number of symptoms and signs can indicate an injury that involves the facial bones including blood in the airway; swellings, depressions, and/or large bruises on the face; deformity of the visual shape of the face; loose or knocked out teeth, broken dentures, or other dental appliances; a swollen lower jaw (along the bone or at its joints); and poor lower-jaw function.

There is little that you can do to provide direct care for a facial fracture. You should, however, make certain that someone alerts the EMS system, keep the athlete at rest, maintain an open airway, control bleeding (do not apply pressure over the site of a possible fracture or

a dislocated lower jaw), treat for shock, and care for soft tissue injuries. Remember to reassure the athlete throughout care.

Care for Lower-Jaw Fracture or Dislocation

Direct blows to the jaw may produce fractures or dislocations. The typical symptoms and signs include pain, swelling, discoloration, malalignment of teeth, facial deformity, and the loss of use. Skeletal injury to the jaw bone or its movable joints often produces difficulties with speech. In most cases, you will not need to provide support for the injured jaw, but you should simply render basic care and wait for the EMTs to arrive.

When an EMS response will be delayed, you can use cravats (3-inch-wide cloth strips) to help support the jaw. This will make the athlete more comfortable. Do *not* tie the athlete's mouth shut! If you do and the athlete vomits, it is possible for him or her to aspirate the vomitus. Alert the EMS system, keep the athlete at rest, maintain an open airway, assess and care for more serious problems (e.g., spinal injury), and then, if appropriate, provide support for the lower jaw.

Application of this support requires you to place the center of a 3-inch-wide cravat slightly above the athlete's left ear. Carry one end of the cravat over the top of the head and the other end under the jaw. Use a half-knot (allows for easier removal in emergencies) to tie

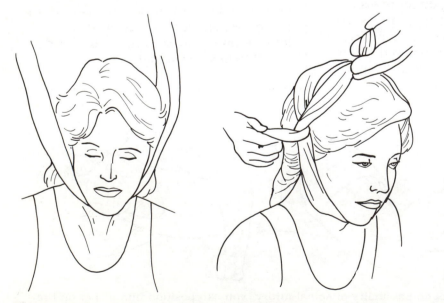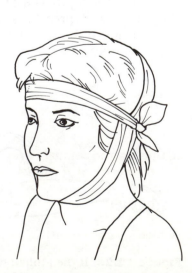

Figure 12.3. Using a cravat for support of a lower jaw injury.

the two ends together at a point slightly above the right ear. Pull one end of the cravat around the back of the head and the other end across the forehead. Knot the two ends above the left ear (see Figure 12.3). Treat for shock and continue to monitor the athlete for vomiting and changes in vital signs and state of awareness.

WARNING:

Do *not* attempt to correct (reduce) a dislocated jaw, even if this is a chronic problem.

Nasal Bone Fractures

The most commonly fractured facial bones are the two nasal bones forming the bridge at the top of the nose. The damage to these bones and the nasal cartilage are often considered to be minor injuries by the layperson, but this is not always the case. More serious injuries may be hidden, and the chance for an infection that could become very serious is always possible. You must ensure an open airway, control bleeding, care for soft-tissue injuries, and make certain that the athlete is treated by a physician. There may be hidden facial fractures that could become the site of a life-threatening infection.

THE SPINE

The spinal column, or backbone, consists of the bones of the neck and the back that create the long-axis support for the body. It serves as the point of attachment for the head, shoulders, ribs, and pelvis. The spinal column houses and protects the spinal cord. A large number of major nerves pass in and out of the spinal cord between the bones of the spine.

The spinal column is made up of 33 bones called vertebrae. These bones are connected by ligaments and separated by disks of cartilage. The structure of the spine allows for flexion, extension, and some rotation and side bending, but highly restricts hyperextension.

The five divisions of the spine include the following (see Figure 12.4):

- *Cervical.* These, the first seven vertebrae, are the neck bones. Most serious sport-

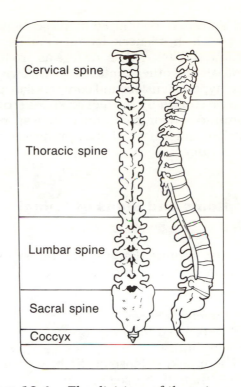

Figure 12.4.   The divisions of the spine.

related spinal injuries involve this region of the spine.
- *Thoracic.* The next 12 vertebrae are the upper-back vertebrae, to which the ribs attach.
- *Lumbar.* The next five vertebrae are the back bones of the lower back.
- *Sacral.* The next five vertebrae are fused together to form the sacrum and are found in the lower back. The pelvis attaches to the sacrum.
- *Coccygeal.* The last four vertebrae are fused together to form the tailbone.

Spinal injuries may take the form of fractures, dislocations, ligament sprains, or disk damage. Most sport-related injuries of the back involve only soft tissues (muscles and ligaments) and do not involve the structures of the spinal column, cord, or nerves. The vertebrae, spinal cord, and nerves are so well protected that they are only injured when improper technique (e.g., spearing in football) is utilized or the individual sustains a catastrophic blow or fall (e.g., gymnastics, diving, pole vaulting). In most cases in which the spine is involved, the injury is a reversible form of tissue swelling. When this occurs, improper initial care may cause more serious injury.

The spine can be injured by direct blows to the top of the head, neck, lateral shoulders and arms, chest, back, pelvis, or legs as produced in football and other contact sports. Twisting forces, hyperextension, and compression along the spine caused by the feet or knees striking the ground or floor, common in such sports as basketball and volleyball, may produce serious spinal injury.

Symptoms and Signs of Spinal Injury

You must assume that a spinal injury exists whenever a force has caused any of the following:

- Unconsciousness
- Severe head injury
- Neck injury
- The breaking loose of the breastbone or ribs (flail chest: see p. 139)
- Possible pelvic fracture
- Possible hip dislocation
- Thigh fracture
- Arm-bone fracture (rarely related to sport injuries)

Often spinal injury can occur without any clear symptoms or signs. In many cases, standard field tests for spinal injury have proven inadequate. For these reasons, the mechanism of injury and the detection of other injuries that are related to spinal damage must be given strong consideration during the assessment. Accidents in diving, skiing, sledding, gymnastics (falls and straddling falls), bicycling, and pole vaulting have the greatest potential for generating forces that can cause spinal injury. Spinal injuries as the result of contact in football do occur, and the injury is usually to the cervical spine.

Assess the athlete for potential spinal injury if you note these symptoms:

- Unconsciousness following injury
- Any injuries that are associated with spinal injuries
- Weakness or paralysis to the arms or legs
- Numbness or tingling sensations in the extremities
- Pain, tenderness, or point tenderness along the back of the neck
- Pain or tenderness along the back

- Burning sensations anywhere along the spine or in an extremity
- Pain along the spine induced by moving an arm or leg (Do not request the athlete to move a limb.)
- Loss of bowel and/or bladder control
- Difficult breathing, where chest movements are limited or absent (Only small abdominal movements can be associated with breathing.)
- Cervical injury positioning (see Figure 12.5) in which the athlete will be down with the arms stretched out over the head or across the chest
- Deformity felt along the spine (rare) or the head at an unusual angle (Do not move the athlete to access deformity.)
- Persistent erection (priapism), indicating a possible spinal injury that has affected (at least) the nerves to the genitals

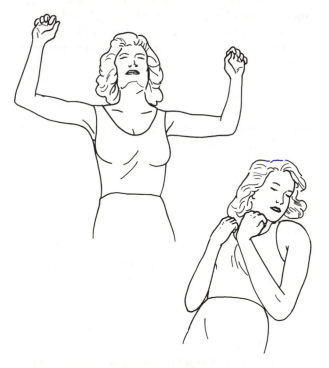

Figure 12.5. Body position indicating the probability of an injury to the cervical spine.

Care for Spinal Injuries

Spinal injuries require you to apply the primary rule of emergency care—*do no harm.* If you take the wrong actions, serious injury or death may result. In providing care for possible spinal injuries, you should take the following steps:

1. Protect the athlete by stopping all nearby activities.
2. Make certain that someone is alerting the EMS system.
3. Provide an open airway using the jaw-thrust technique and rescue breathing or CPR if required.
4. Control all life-threatening bleeding.
5. Keep the athlete at rest. Do not move the athlete, reposition his or her body or any of its parts, or attempt to splint fractures. Any movement of the limbs may cause additional severe injury along the spine. Reassure the athlete and explain the importance of remaining still.
6. Stabilize the athlete's head, neck, and as much of the body as possible. Kneel at the athlete's head and gently hold (do not lift) the head along the sides of the face (see Figure 12.6). Do not apply any tension to the head or neck.

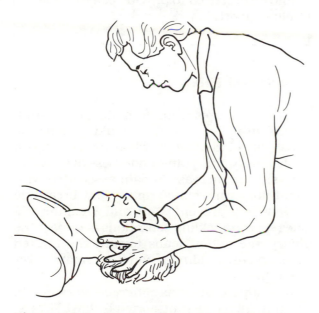

Figure 12.6. In case of possible head, neck, or back injuries, stabilize the athlete's head.

7. Cover the athlete to begin treating for shock. Do not allow the athlete to become overheated.
8. Constantly monitor the athlete for changes in breathing and pulse. Stay alert for vomiting. Do not turn the athlete's head to clear vomitus. The body must be turned as a single unit to a position on the side.

> **WARNING:**
>
> Do *not* apply a soft cervical collar. This device is of little use in emergency care. A rigid cervical, or extrication, collar is needed to provide the necessary support. Application of these collars requires specialized training. Do *not* place the athlete onto a long spine board. An extrication collar *must* be applied before the athlete can be moved to a spine board. The proper technique for repositioning and securing the athlete to a long spine board is a specialized skill.

Possible Disk Injuries

Most sport-related problems with the disks occur to the lumbar disks. The second-most common location is the cervical spine. Damage to the lumbar disk may be expressed by back pain with pain radiating from the back into one or both extremities, a burning sensation in the back and/or down the lower extremities, and restricted movement. When a cervical disk is injured, there may be pain in the neck, pain radiating down one or both upper limbs, restriction of head movements, and numbness or tingling sensations in the neck or upper extremities.

Any athlete with indications of possible disk injury should be examined by a physician. If the symptoms and signs occur after an impact or activity, keep the athlete at rest and request an EMS response as there could be more serious injuries. In addition, simple movement and activities could cause additional damage to the disk, nerves, or spinal cord. If the problem is reported the next day or several days after an activity or has a sudden onset following a simple activity such as bending over to tie a shoe, the athlete should consult a physician. The athlete may either have a simple case of strain, the indications of more serious injury, or the first sign of a spinal disease. In cases in which the pain is severe, range of motion is limited, or walking is restricted, arrange for EMS transport.

Fractured Coccyx

A hard fall to the buttocks or lower back may produce a fractured coccyx. The athlete will have pain and possibly tenderness at the site, but there should be no other indications of spinal or pelvic injury. Although the fracture should heal unattended, the athlete must see a physician to confirm a fractured coccyx, to be certain that the injury is limited to the coccyx and surrounding soft tissues, and to receive instructions for proper and complete healing. The athlete must not be allowed to participate in sport activities until cleared by the attending physician.

THE CHEST

The vital organs, blood vessels, and nerves of the chest are protected by the ribs. The lower ribs offer some protection for the stomach, spleen, gall bladder, and liver. There are 12 ribs on each side of the chest, and all 12 pairs attach in the back to the thoracic vertebrae.

Starting at the top, the first seven pairs attach in the front of the body directly to the breastbone (sternum) by way of cartilage. The next three pairs of ribs attach in the front to the cartilage that connects the seventh rib to the breastbone. The lower two pairs of ribs are called floating ribs. They have no attachments to the cartilage of the ribs above them or to the breastbone (see Figure 12.7).

Most skeletal injuries of the chest involve the ribs. When a rib is fractured, there is usually no serious damage to any internal organs, although a very forceful impact may fracture several ribs and/or the breastbone. The first four pairs of ribs are seldom fractured in sport-related injuries because they are too well protected by the bones and muscles of the shoulder girdle and upper back. The movement of

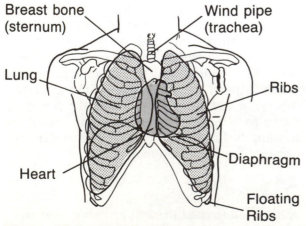

Breast bone (sternum)

Wind pipe (trachea)

Lung

Ribs

Heart

Diaphragm

Floating Ribs

Figure 12.7. The rib cage.

the floating ribs (because of their lack of frontal attachments) helps reduce the frequency of fractures of these ribs. Sport-injury-related rib fractures tend to occur to the fifth through the tenth pairs of ribs.

WARNING:

Severe injuries to the ribs or breastbone may cause injury to the lungs and the heart. If the athlete has frothy red blood in the mouth or is coughing up this blood, the lungs are probably punctured (see below). The athlete has a life-threatening condition if you detect severe problems with breathing; a blue coloration to the skin of the head, neck, and shoulders; blue coloration and swelling of the lips and tongue; bulging and bloodshot eyes; bulging neck veins; deviation of the trachea from center; or an obvious chest deformity. Constantly monitor the athlete and be prepared to provide basic cardiac life support.

Fractured Ribs

Most rib fractures result from direct force that occurs during impact. You should consider the possibility of rib fracture when you detect pain at the injury site, point tenderness over the injury site, an increase in pain associated with breathing or movement or shallow breathing (to reduce or prevent pain), and when the athlete reports crackling sensations at or near the injury site and/or leans toward the injured side, usually holding a hand or forearm over the injury site.

Any athlete who has suffered a possible rib fracture should be transported by the EMS system to a medical facility to make certain that the injury is limited to a simple rib fracture and to receive any necessary care. If only one or two ribs are fractured, you need to keep the athlete at rest until the EMTs arrive. A sling and swathe can be applied. Contrary to the popular practice, do not tape the chest.

You must consider the injury to be very serious if the athlete shows any indications of breathing problems or injured lungs. Coughing up frothy red blood is a strong indication of such injury. Have someone alert the EMS system while you begin to treat the athlete for shock.

Flail Chest

When a rib is fractured in two places, it may act independently from the rest of the chest wall. If three or more consecutive ribs on the same side of the chest are fractured in two places, a significant portion of the chest wall will not move with the rest of the chest during respirations. In fact, the section will appear to be moving in a direction opposite that of the rest of the chest wall (paradoxical respirations). This condition is called a *flail chest* and differs from a rib fracture (see Figure 12.8). The same condition can be produced when the breastbone is fractured away from the ribs. A flail chest can be life threatening to the victim.

The athlete is considered to have a flail chest when you find the symptoms and signs of a rib fracture and a section of the chest wall that fails to move with the rest of the wall when the athlete breathes. *Consider a flail chest to be a life-threatening emergency.* You should take the following steps (see Figure 12.9):

1. Stop all activity around the athlete.
2. Keep the athlete at rest and make certain there is an open airway.
3. Have someone alert the EMS system.
4. Expose the injury site by cutting away clothing.
5. Place a thick pad of dressing (several inches thick) or a small pillow over the injury site.
6. Use large strips of tape or cravats to hold the pad in place. This will help to stabilize the flailed section of the chest

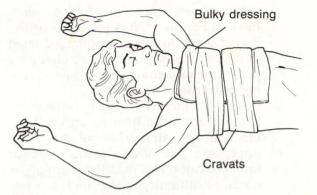

Figure 12.9. Care for flail chest.

wall. If these these methods will not hold, use your hand to keep the pad in place (do not apply too much pressure) or have the athlete lie on the injured side.
7. Treat for shock.
8. Monitor the airway, breathing, and pulse.

SUMMARY AND RECOMMENDATIONS

Remember that injuries to the head, spine, and chest may render the athlete unconscious. Always assume that the unconscious injured athlete has spinal injuries. Protect him or her from the elements and ensure eye protection.

1. A severe head injury may directly or indirectly damage the brain. Indirect brain injuries include concussions and brain bruises (contusions).
2. A brain injury may have occurred if the athlete has any signs of skull fracture. Brain injury is possible if the athlete is

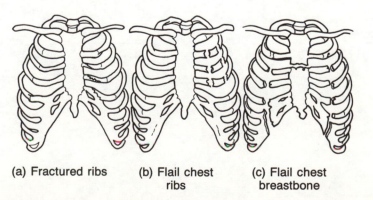

(a) Fractured ribs (b) Flail chest ribs (c) Flail chest breastbone

Figure 12.8. A comparison of (a) a rib fracture, (b) a flail chest (rib), and (c) a flail chest (breastbone).

unconscious, suffers from loss of awareness, is confused, has paralysis or the loss of sensation, has unequally dilated or unresponsive pupils, has a changing pulse rate and character, or has changing patterns of respiration.

3. Consider a facial fracture to be possible if there are large bruises on the face, blood in the airway, facial deformity (including the lower jaw), loose or knocked-out teeth, malalignment of the teeth, or difficulty using the lower jaw (including difficulty with speech). Make certain there is an open airway. Apply basic care for soft-tissue injuries and treat for shock.

4. Spinal injuries can be difficult to assess. Assume there is spinal injury if the injured athlete is unconscious, has suffered a severe injury to the head, neck, shoulder and upper arm (rarely related to sport injuries), chest, pelvis, hip, or thigh, or pain along the spine. Survey for spinal injury, taking special note of weakness, numbness, tingling, or paralysis. While waiting for an EMS response, do not move or reposition the athlete but stabilize the head and neck, treat for shock (do not lift the legs), and constantly monitor breathing and pulse. Take no actions unless you have been trained to do so. *Do no harm.*

5. Skeletal injury of the chest can include fractured ribs or flail chest. Pain and point tenderness at the injury site are the major signs of rib fracture. In most cases, you can keep the athlete at rest until the EMTs arrive. A flail chest will show the signs of a fractured rib and a section of chest that fails to move with the rest of the chest wall. Secure a thick pad of dressings or a pillow over the injury site. Consider this to be a life-threatening emergency.

Chapter 13
Environmental Factors

A number of factors in the environment can cause problems for the athlete that will require assessment and care. These problems are seen most often in outdoor winter and summer sports. Football, because it is played into the late fall and early winter and is practiced in the summer in some areas, tends to be one of the sports that is affected most by harsh environmental factors.

Most problems due to environmental factors are related to excessive heat or cold. The coach's primary course of action should always be one of *prevention*. A little thought about the potential problems and a little effort to ensure adequate protection for your athletes will eliminate most serious emergencies that are related to environmental factors.

HEAT-RELATED PROBLEMS

Exposure to excessive heat can quickly bring about emergencies, some of which are life threatening. These problems are most often associated with outdoor activities in the summer; however, poorly ventilated, hot indoor facilities can also cause heat emergencies.

It is difficult to define "excessive heat." Each individual has a specific tolerance to heat exposure that may vary depending on general health, level of fitness, acclimatization, state of exhaustion, recent diet, and liquid and salt consumption. For some people exertion in an environment of 80°F can quickly cause heat-related problems. Other individuals can tolerate very high temperatures for long periods of time. Keep a close watch on your athletes so that you can spot exhaustion, cramping, or the shutdown of perspiration.

> **WARNING:**
> Certain over-the-counter preparations may make an athlete more susceptible to heat-related problems. For example, aspirin and antihistamines change sweat patterns. Aspirin causes an increase in sweat loss, and when taken in large doses may cause an increase in body temperature above that resulting from physical activity alone. Antihistamines, on the other hand, decrease the athlete's rate of sweating.

Realize that hot, humid environments are most often associated with heat-related problems, but hot temperatures with low humidity can cause severe reactions. In moist-heat situations, the evaporation of sweat is limited, thus reducing cooling. At temperatures from 80°F to 90°F and a humidity under 70%, there are usually few problems. Once the humidity goes above 70% or the temperature goes above 90°F, you should exercise extreme caution concerning the amount of activity allowed without rest and the replacement of lost liquids and electrolytes. It is often better to change the time of the activity than to allow long participation when the temperature is above 90°F and the humidity over 70%. A temperature above 100°F, even when the humidity is below 70%, may cause severe heat-related problems. Figure 13.1 details specific danger zones.

You can prevent heat-related problems by making certain that you have followed these procedures:

- Your athletes should be properly dressed for exposure to the heat. Having them wear a winter uniform during an August

Relative humidity

Actual temperature (°F)	30%	50%	70%	90%
102	108	125	Heat index	Heat
100	105	120	above 130	index
98	101	110	Heat stroke likely	above 130
96	98	108	128	Heat stroke
94	95	105	122	likely
92	92	100	115	
90	90	96	106	122
88	87	93	100	115
86	85	90	96	109
84	83	86	91	99
82	80	84	89	95
80	78	81	85	89

Apparent temperatures based on the combined effect of actual temperature and relative humidity

- Extreme Danger
- Danger
- Extreme Caution
- Caution

Figure 13.1. Heat index as indicated by the National Weather Service.

practice is asking for trouble. Hot weather uniforms should be loose-fitting and made of cotton.

- Where appropriate, hats should be worn as protection from the sun. When they are not engaged in activity, allow football players to remove their helmets.
- Provide protection from the sun and/or a cool rest spot.
- Water must be available. In hot conditions, you must rest your athletes every 20-30 minutes and have each of them drink 8 ounces of water. Water is recommended for fluid replacement. However, half-strength commercial electrolyte drinks can be used. Be aware, however,

that these and other salted fluids may delay the absorption of needed water. It is best to limit their use to before and after practice. Salt pills should not be given to your athletes.

- Weigh athletes before and after each practice during hot and/or humid months of the season. A loss of 2 pounds reflects the loss of a quart of water. Athletes should report to practice each day at approximately the same weight if they are properly hydrated. Proper hydration is a key to preventing heat-related problems.
- Allow no one to continue participating if they are exhausted or suffering muscle cramps.

• Activity should be reduced if the heat has a sudden onset (e.g., a summer heat wave) or if the athletes have not been conditioned for the heat. It can take 2-3 weeks for most people to acclimatize to activity in heat, with children requiring more time than adults. You should schedule your activities at no more than 30-45 minutes initially, working up to a maximum limit of 2 hours.

WARNING:

Two common practices should be avoided. First, do not make use of salt tablets. Liberal salting of food and appropriate fluid-replacement strategies eliminate the need for these dangerous tablets. Second, do not allow athletes to wear vinyl sweat suits as such attire increases the risk of heat-related injury. Vinyl does not allow the evaporation of sweat, the prime cooling mechanism.

Heat Cramps

Heat cramps are always possible when the athlete is exposed to heat for a long period of time, and the heat does not have to be much greater than a comfortable environmental temperature. Water and salts are lost from the body due to heavy perspiration. Recent medical studies indicate that it is the water loss that will eventually cause severe muscle cramps. You can help prevent heat cramps by providing frequent water breaks during practice and providing an ample water supply during competitions.

As heat cramps develop, the symptoms and signs that develop include leg (usually calf) and/or abdominal muscle cramps, physical exhaustion that may lead to collapse, and dizziness that may lead to fainting (rare). Keep in mind that the development of cramps may be delayed (especially with young athletes), thus making exhaustion and dizziness more reliable signs.

When heat cramps are detected, you should take these steps (see Figure 13.2):

1. Move the athlete to a cool place that is as close to the scene as possible.

2. Give the athlete water to drink. Do *not* give cold water. Muscle cramps should reduce in severity shortly after drinking fluids.

3. Gently massage (do not knead) the cramped muscles. Do not massage the muscles of any athlete who has a history of circulatory problems that have lead to the formation of blood clots in veins. These problems are seen most often in middle and late adulthood and are usually limited to the veins of the lower legs.

4. If needed, apply cool moist towels to the athlete's forehead and over the cramped muscles. In some cases, this will reduce the severity of pain caused by the muscle cramps.

Many EMS systems recommend that they be alerted in *all* cases of heat cramps. Check with your local rescue squad or hospital emergency department to see if this is the policy for your area.

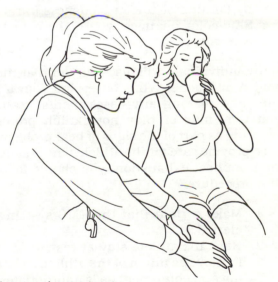

Signs and symptoms:
muscle cramps (legs and abdomen), exhaustion, dizziness or faintness
Care:
• Move to a nearby cool place.
• Give salted water to drink, or half-strength comercial electrolyte fluids.
• Massage the cramped muscle.
• Apply moist towels to forehead and over cramped muscles.
• If cramps continue, or if more serious signs and symptoms develop, alert EMS system.

Figure 13.2. Care of heat cramps.

Heat Exhaustion

Heat exhaustion results from excessive heat exposure and loss of fluid and leads to blood collecting near the skin in an effort to release heat. As expected, it is seen most often during the summer months, when the athlete is exposed to excessive heat while exercising or while participating in an event. The amount of activity does not have to be that strenuous. Sometimes, heat exhaustion occurs during indoor activity where the temperature may be high and the ventilation poor.

The athlete who is suffering from heat exhaustion will display some or all these symptoms and signs:

- Rapid and shallow breathing
- A weak pulse (sometimes described as very thready)
- Heavy perspiration that usually produces a cool and clammy skin
- Exhaustion that leads to the athlete saying that he or she feels weak
- Dizziness that sometimes may be followed by fainting or unconsciousness (rare)
- Skin-color changes where the skin becomes pale

Many individuals will also tell you that they have a headache. While observing your athletes and making any assessments, realize that they may or may not exhibit profuse sweating as part of the signs of heat problems.

To provide care for the athlete who is suffering from heat exhaustion, you should follow this procedure:

1. Make certain that the EMS system is alerted.
2. Have the athlete stay at rest.
3. Remove as much of the athlete's clothing and equipment as is appropriate to allow for body cooling. Do *not* allow the athlete to become chilled. Fan the athlete to promote cooling.
4. Provide the conscious athlete with water. In addition, half-strength commercial electrolytes or salted water (1 teaspoon of salt in 3 quarts of water) can be provided to help replenish lost salts. *Do not give fluids to the unconscious athlete.* Do not delay providing the athlete with water to drink so that you can find or make a salted drink.
5. Start to treat the athlete for shock. Make certain that you cover the athlete *but not to the point of overheating* (use a lightweight sheet, not a blanket). Overheating at this stage may cause abnormal heart activity to develop rapidly.

WARNING:

In cases of possible heat exhaustion in which the athlete becomes unconscious or fails to recover quickly or there is a history of medical problems or recent injury, you can expect the athlete's condition to worsen.

Heat Stroke

There is no such thing as a case of heat stroke that is not serious. Heat stroke is a *true emergency* that can quickly lead to severe brain damage or death. All cases of heat stroke require an EMS response so that the athlete can be taken to a medical facility as quickly as possible.

In most cases, heat stroke occurs when the athlete who is exposed to excessive heat stops sweating. This is not an absolute for all cases. Heat stroke usually occurs on a hot and humid day, but dry heat can cause the same problem. The common name for heat stroke is *sunstroke*, which often leads one to believe that collapse due to exposure to the sun is less serious than heat stroke. Regardless of the source of excessive heat, heat stroke is always a true emergency.

Heat stroke will produce varying symptoms and signs that usually include the following:

- A period of deep breathing followed by rapid and shallow breathing
- Initially, a rapid and strong pulse that changes to a rapid and weak one
- Dry, hot skin
- A reddening of the skin (sometimes)
- Dilated pupils
- Faintness
- Dizziness
- Headache
- Nausea
- Eventual unconsciousness
- Convulsions or twitching (sometimes)

It is important to remember that heat stroke can occur without heat cramps, heat exhaustion, or other observable heat-related problem developing first.

To provide care for the athlete who may have heat stroke, you should take these steps (see Figure 13.3):

1. Make certain that someone alerts the EMS system. Do not delay cooling the athlete so that you can make the call.
2. Cool the athlete as rapidly as possible. Any delay could lead to brain damage and death. If the emergency occurs outside, move the athlete out of the sun (the shade must be nearby) or have others quickly construct a sunshield (by using blankets) as you continue with care. Remove the athlete's equipment and clothing and provide a wrap of wet towels and sheets. Continue to pour water over the wrap. This water should be as cool as is readily available. Use tepid water for preschool age children.
3. Continue to cool the athlete rapidly by using ice packs or cold packs. These should be wrapped and placed where large blood vessels are close to the surface of the skin, including the sides of the neck, the armpits, the wrists, the ankles, and the groin. Once these are in place, continue to fan the athlete.
4. Continue to monitor pulse and respiration and be prepared to provide basic cardiac life support.
5. Continue to apply cool water to the wrappings to lower the athlete's body temperature.

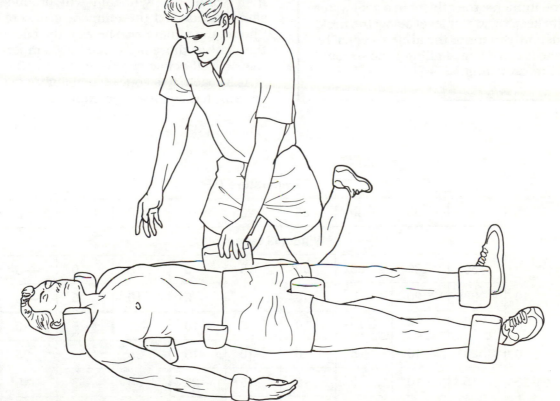

Signs and symptoms:
deep breaths often followed by shallow breathing; rapid pulse; dry, hot skin; dilated pupils; loss of consciousness; convulsions or twitching
Care:

• Wrap cold packs or ice backs. Place one under each armpit, wrist, and ankle; on each side of the athlete's neck; and at the groin.

• If transport is delayed and permission granted by a physician, immerse up to face in cooled water and monitor constantly to prevent drowning.
• Monitor pulse and breathing.
• Treat for shock.

Figure 13.3. Care of heat stroke.

Once the cooling of the athlete is under way, have someone place a second call to the EMS dispatcher to find out if there will be a long delay before help arrives. If there will be, have the caller ask if you should place the athlete in cool water. Even when there is going to be a delay, the recommendation for a cool-water soaking usually will not be given. This is because research has shown that cool-water baths often greatly reduce circulation to the skin, allowing for a rapid buildup of heat in deep tissues, increased body temperature, and the chances of brain damage due to excessive heat. A cool-water bath should only be administered on the recommendation of the EMS system or a physician.

WARNING:

If you immerse the athlete in a cool-water bath, keep the water level below the neck. Constantly monitor the athlete even if he or she is conscious. Failing to do so could lead to drowning.

COLD-RELATED PROBLEMS

For some individuals, the environmental temperature does not have to be too far below the comfort range before they start to react to cold. This is especially true for the very young and old and for people who have chronic illnesses or who have sustained injuries. As the environmental temperature falls, even the typical individual will begin to react to the cold, often being unaware of this reaction in its initial stages.

The effects of cold can be accelerated by water and wind. Coaches must consider the cold environment to be more significant if the athlete becomes soaked with perspiration, rain, or water from another source.

The windchill factor must be watched closely. For example, if the actual temperature on a playing field is 25°F and there is a 15-mile-per-hour wind, the windchill will produce the same effects as if the temperature were 0°F. Should the athlete also be wet, the effects are the same as those produced by a temperature that is well below zero (see Figure 13.4).

As a coach, it is your responsibility to make certain that adequate precautions have been

	Temperature (°F)								
Calm	40	35	30	25	20	15	10	5	0
	Windchill temperature								
5	35	30	25	20	15	10	5	0	−5
10	30	20	15	10	5	0	−10	−15	−20
15	25	15	10	0	−5	−10	−20	−25	−30
20	20	10	5	0	−10	−15	−25	−30	−35
25	15	10	0	−5	−15	−20	−30	−35	−45
30	10	5	0	−10	−20	−25	−30	−40	−50
35	10	5	−5	−10	−20	−30	−35	−40	−50
40	10	0	−5	−15	−20	−30	−35	−45	−55

Wind speed (mph)

Flesh may freeze within one minute.

Figure 13.4. Equivalent windchill temperatures as indicated by the National Weather Service.

taken to protect your athletes from excessive cold. These steps may include the following:

- Providing a warm rest area for the athletes
- Utilizing uniforms that are designed for the environmental temperature
- Having uniform changes available in case the athlete becomes wet or is soaked with perspiration
- Having the athletes use the proper protective gear, including head and hand protection
- Providing blankets for periods of inactivity
- Keeping athletes who are not participating from remaining inactive for too long a period of time
- Resting athletes who show minor skin reactions to cold exposure (see the discussion on frostnip below) or breathing problems caused by cold-air exposure
- Reducing the time of exposure if the cold has a sudden onset or if the athletes are not conditioned for the cold

Frostnip

Frostnip is local cooling, which most frequently affects the tip of the nose, the earlobes, the tips of the fingers, and the upper cheeks. Although frostnip is not serious and the athlete will respond quickly to care, you should not forget that this reaction to cold is a form of frostbite. Think of frostnip as an early warning that signifies that a more serious form of frostbite is likely to develop unless specific action is taken.

The symptoms and signs used to assess frostnip have a slow onset and development. The affected skin will become lighter in pigmentation (usually blanching, or turning white), and the frostnipped part will feel numb to the athlete. The athlete is usually unaware of the problem and often requires someone to tell him or her that the skin color has changed.

The athlete can care for his or her own case of frostnip by placing frostnipped fingers in the armpits to provide the needed warmth or by the simple act of blowing warm air on the site. Other affected areas can be cared for by covering the site with the hands. The athlete may report tingling or burning sensations during the rewarming process.

WARNING:
If the frostnipped area does not respond to simple care, assume that the athlete has a more serious form of frostbite and treat accordingly.

Superficial Frostbite

Superficial frostbite is the condition that most people call "frostbite." All cases of superficial frostbite must be considered serious since tissues have been damaged by the formation of ice crystals in the skin, and if it is allowed to go untreated, tissue death may occur. If enough tissue cells die, the affected limb may be lost or the person may die.

The two most noticeable signs of frostbite include

- the frostbitten area becoming pale, usually appearing white and waxy; and
- the affected area feeling frozen at the skin surface but retaining its normal softness and elasticity (bounce) below the surface.

If the affected area feels frozen below the skin surface, assume that you are dealing with a case of freezing. The field emergency care will be the same as for superficial frostbite.

The care for superficial frostbite includes taking the following steps:

1. Make certain that the EMS system is alerted.
2. Protect the affected area—the frostbitten site should be covered and handled as *gently* as possible.
3. Apply warmth to the site—the source of the heat should be a steady one and the temperature should be comfortable enough to be held in one's bare hand. The source can be hot-water bottles filled with warm water, another person's body heat, or heat packs (see pp. 187-188) with enough wrapping to reduce the temperature to between 100°F and 105°F (comfortable enough to hold).
4. Keep the athlete warm and at rest. Do *not* allow the athlete to walk on a frostbitten foot.

If the EMS response will be delayed, rewarm the frostbitten part by immersing it in a container of warm water, unless there is a chance it could refreeze before help arrives. The ideal temperature range for this water is from 100°F to 105°F. The water must be at a temperature that produces no discomfort when you place your finger in it. As much of the injured part as possible should be immersed without touching the bottom or the sides of the container. During rewarming, you should remove some of the water as it cools and replace it with warm water.

As the frostbitten part rewarms, the athlete will experience some pain. This is a good sign as it indicates the reduction of ice crystals and improved circulation in the affected area. Severe frostbite will usually produce severe pain during the rewarming process.

Rewarming is complete once the affected part no longer feels frozen and begins to turn red or blue. At this point, you should dry the area and wrap it in a clean dressing. If the affected part is a hand or foot, you should place pads of dressing between the fingers or toes prior to applying the dressing wrap.

After dressing the affected part, cover it with blankets, towels, or clothing to help maintain its warmth. Elevate any limb that has a frostbitten part. Continue to keep the athlete at rest and as warm as possible without overheating.

WARNING:

Do *not* rub a frostbitten body part. Do *not* rub snow on the injury site. Any rough handling of the frostbitten part may cause severe tissue damage. Do *not* rewarm a frostbitten part if there is a chance that it will refreeze before EMS help arrives.

SUN PROTECTION

Maximum skin protection from solar exposure is part of safe sport participation. Not only is sunburn protection important, but it is part of a coach's responsibility to warn athletes of the dangers of skin damage and cancer that result from overexposure to harmful solar ultraviolet radiation. The coach must point out that the

major purpose of participation is not to improve one's tan. Overexposure to the sun is dangerous for everyone, including children and young adults.

The coach must make certain that the athlete is protected by the uniform that is suitable for practice and participation. Male athletes should be instructed not to take off their shirts during practice or while waiting to participate. When it is necessary to protect bare skin, commercial sunscreen (sunblock) with a skin protection factor-15 rating or higher should be applied. The athletes should not be allowed to apply homemade screens, baby oil, or suntan lotions as these compounds may offer little protection against harmful radiation.

WARNING:

Certain common prescription drugs, such as tetracyclene or sulfa drugs, cause an individual to be more sensitive to ultraviolet rays, and therefore more likely to burn.

AIR POLLUTION

Poor air quality and smog can present real dangers to the athlete. Both short and long-term lung damage are possible from participating in unsafe air. It is true that participating in clean air is not possible in many localities, but restricting activity is recommended when the air-quality ratings are worse than moderate or when there is a smog alert. Your local health department or air-quality control board can inform you of the air-quality ratings for your area and when restricting activities is recommended.

Do not be fooled into believing that you must be in a large city to be concerned about air quality. Many small towns are subject to poor air quality from motor-vehicle emissions that are trapped by temperature inversions or natural barriers (e.g., mountains). Additional problems may occur when the air is still and pollutants from factories settle in valleys. Even agricultural spraying may cause temporary air-quality problems.

Your decision to allow participation must be based on air-quality reports and the recommendations of local health agencies and physicians. It is suggested that your school or local department of recreation have a medical advisor to supply its coaches with guidelines and to offer specific warnings as to when to restrict or halt participation.

SUMMARY AND RECOMMENDATIONS

1. Most problems caused by the hot and/or humid environment can be avoided through preventive measures that are designed to reduce exposure and ensure proper fluid replacement.
2. The most common problems associated with excessive heat are heat cramps, heat exhaustion, and heat stroke. These problems can be avoided if your ath-

letes are slowly conditioned to play in the heat (not above 90°F if the humidity is above 70% and not above 100°F even at low humidity), adequate rest periods with the necessary protection are provided, and fluids are given.
3. The proper clothing and protection from the cold must be given to athletes to prevent serious problems caused by low temperatures. Frostnip is a limited, local cooling that the athlete can correct by using his or her own body heat to rewarm the affected part. Frostbite requires an EMS response because ice crystals have formed in the skin.
4. Provide warnings to athletes about the dangers of overexposure to the sun's rays and take action to limit the effects.
5. Be aware of air-quality conditions in your area and curtail participation in athletic events as necessary.

Chapter 14
Medical Problems and Emergencies

The coach must have a basic knowledge of the illnesses that cause emergency situations to arise during sport participation. The preseason physical examination, following physicians' instructions, and properly assessing possible emergencies will help you decide on the proper care to be given.

Most chronic medical problems will be uncovered and/or noted during the preseason physical. You can use this information to prepare for certain types of problems and to know how to help the athlete. For example, you may have an athlete who is subject to asthma attacks as a result of exercise and/or stress. For this athlete you should have specific directions for rest or for taking prescribed medications and resting.

Undetected chronic problems, as well as new problems that have a sudden onset (acute problems), may cause an emergency that requires immediate initial care. Some of these problems may prove to be life threatening. Through interviews with the athlete and bystanders and by applying a few simple examination techniques such as determining pulse and breathing rates, assessing relative skin temperature, and feeling for the indications of abdominal tenderness, the coach can detect many possible emergencies and problems that require immediate attention, such as heart attacks, respiratory distress, acute abdomen, and various infectious diseases.

When dealing with emergencies and problems, your role will not be to diagnose and treat. Instead, you will be trying to *detect the presence of a possible medical problem*, not the specific problem. Once this is determined, your next course of action is to (a) provide the needed initial care, (b) make certain that an EMS response is made, or (c) make sure that the athlete sees the proper health care professional.

Certain symptoms and signs help to determine the existence of a possible problem and whether that problem presents an emergency. From your own experiences you know that, for example, fever, nausea, aches and pains, vomiting, and diarrhea indicate the possibility of a medical problem. You must learn to associate what you know about illness to the assessment in terms of the interview, gathering of vital signs, and specific steps in the physical examination.

THE HEART

The preseason physical has perhaps its greatest value in determining potential problems with the heart. For the child and young athlete, these are usually related to defects of the heart present at birth or due to childhood infectious diseases (e.g., streptococcal infections). The athlete's medical history and the preseason physical exam can detect most of these problems. This knowledge can be used by the physician to channel the athlete into a sport in which he or she can be successful even with the cardiac condition.

The athlete's medical history may suggest that you restrict certain activities. The athlete's age should increase your awareness for potential heart attacks. Regardless of the athlete's age and medical history, you must suspect heart problems if any of the following occur:

- *Chest pain.* This may occur under the breastbone and start in the chest and spread to the shoulder or start in the chest and spread down one arm. The athlete may hold a fist over the pain site on the chest. The pain will not be a small spot of "stabbing" pain or simply sharp twinges of pain but is usually a steady pain of marked discomfort involving an area of the chest at least the size of the athlete's fist. In some cases, the pain will not be in the chest but may be in the arm or lower jaw.

- *Chest discomfort*. The athlete may report a tightness or squeezing sensation in the chest. Sometimes this may be described as pressure or a feeling of fullness. Even if the athlete has a history of asthma or other breathing problems related to allergies, you cannot rule out an impending heart attack.
- *Shortness of breath*. Breathing will be labored and usually shallow and rapid.
- *Profuse sweating*.
- *Weakness*.
- *Nausea*.
- *Restlessness*. Although the athlete is not feeling well, he or she will want to stand and walk around or perhaps exercise and may become combative.
- *Fear*. The athlete will have a feeling of impending doom, which may make the athlete deny pain or discomfort.

To provide care for an athlete who may be having, or who may be about to have, a heart attack, you should do the following:

1. *Stay calm*. You must carry out all the steps of care in a calm, professional manner to help reduce the athlete's anxiety.
2. *Make certain that someone alerts the EMS system*. This person should tell the dispatcher what you have observed. In some localities, the dispatcher will send a cardiac life support unit. Do not leave the athlete to place the call yourself as cardiac arrest could occur while you are away.
3. *Reassure the athlete*. It is critical that the athlete relax as much as possible. Your emotional support could prove to be a key element in the athlete's survival. If the athlete asks if he or she is having a heart attack, simply state that the problem could be due to a lot of things, but no chances will be taken.

4. *Keep the athlete at rest in a comfortable position*. Help the athlete to assume a position that allows for easy breathing. Most often this is a semi-sitting position. Do *not* let the athlete exert him- or herself; rather, you should reposition the athlete.
5. *Loosen any restrictive equipment or clothing and cover the athlete to prevent chill*. It is critical that you do not overheat the athlete.
6. *Monitor the athlete's pulse and breathing*. Be prepared to initiate CPR if necessary.

WARNING:

If there are any indications that the athlete may be having, or is about to have, a heart attack, you *must* provide care as if a heart attack is taking place.

RESPIRATORY DISTRESS

Many factors can cause a person to suffer respiratory distress. An allergy may irritate and swell respiratory membranes, thus limiting the flow of air. Mucus secreted during an infection may partially obstruct the exchange of air. Chronic diseases and conditions such as asthma or bronchitis may cause problems that lead to respiratory distress.

Most respiratory distress cases will produce the following signs:

- Difficult or labored breathing
- Rapid or slowed breathing rate
- Rapid or slowed pulse rate with unusual character
- Unusual breathing sounds

In addition, severe cases might produce the following:

- Changes in skin, lip, or nail-bed color (blue or gray)
- A low level of awareness, confusion, or unconsciousness

Most cases of respiratory distress require you to take the following steps:

1. Make certain that the EMS system is alerted. Do not leave the athlete as conditions may worsen and respiratory arrest is possible.
2. Make certain that an open airway is maintained and keep checking for possible airway obstructions.
3. Be certain that the problem is not due to an allergy. Is a substance causing the allergic reaction at the scene? If it is, can this substance be removed, or can the athlete be moved away from the substance?
4. Keep the athlete at rest and in a position that allows easy breathing (See Figure 14.1).
5. Loosen any restrictive equipment or clothing.
6. Cover the athlete to conserve body heat but avoid overheating.
7. If the athlete appears to have an excess of mucus in the airway that is making breathing difficult or that causes coughing, you should encourage the athlete to cough.
8. Monitor vital signs.
9. Provide emotional support and take the necessary steps to reduce stress.

In most cases, respiratory distress will correct itself; however, you cannot predict when this will or will not occur. Likewise, you will not be able to predict when a case of respiratory distress will apparently correct itself and then immediately recur in an equal or a more severe form. Request EMS support unless you know that you are dealing with a simple problem caused by overexertion while suffering from a minor respiratory problem (e.g., "getting over a cold") or hyperventilation without any complications or signs of other problems.

Hyperventilation

The athlete who is hyperventilating will be breathing too rapidly and too deeply. This is usually a minor problem that has been caused by stress or fear. However, hyperventilation may be a sign of a more serious problem such as an impending heart attack or severe respiratory distress. If the athlete does not respond immediately to your efforts to correct the hyperventilation or if there are signs of another medical problem, alert the EMS system.

A hyperventilating person will have rapid breathing and pulse rate and will sometimes report tingling sensations in the arms and cramps in the fingers. Sharp chest pains may occur, but they will be unlike those of an impending heart attack. If skin-color changes develop, producing the blue or grey color of cyanosis, assume that there is a more serious problem that will require an EMS response.

The rapid breathing that takes place during an attack of hyperventilation will lower the concentration of carbon dioxide in the blood; control of the attack requires that this level be brought back to near-normal levels by having the athlete breathe into a paper bag (do not use plastic; see Figure 14.2). Rebreathing his or her own air will increase the carbon dioxide level and stop the hyperventilation. If this does not work, call for an EMS response. After a simple attack of hyperventilation, rest the athlete and make sure that someone watches for other signs to develop or for hyperventilation to recur. If either occurs, alert the EMS system.

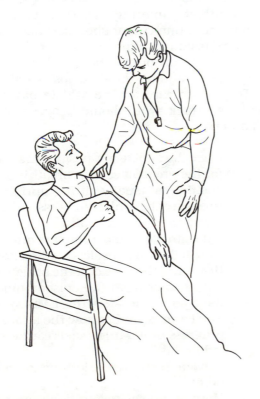

Figure 14.1. Positioning of an athlete to allow for easy breathing.

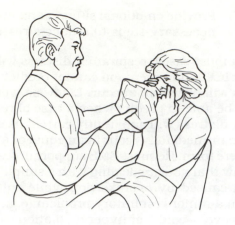

Figure 14.2. You can alleviate hyperventilation by having the athlete breathe into a paper bag.

Spontaneous Pneumothorax

One form of respiratory distress has been associated with young males in their late teens or early twenties who are described as being thin and "athletic." This form of respiratory distress is called *spontaneous pneumothorax*. It has a sudden onset and produces sharp chest pains prior to breathing distress. Apparently, a weakened section of the lung ruptures and releases air into the chest cavity. Breathing will usually be rapid and difficult, and the pulse will become weak. In some cases, the trachea will deviate to one side of the neck, and the chest wall may bulge outward between the ribs and above the collarbone. All cases of spontaneous pneumothorax are life threatening and require an immediate EMS response.

Chronic Pulmonary Diseases

Many chronic pulmonary diseases will disqualify the athlete from participation; however, some conditions—especially asthma—may be present and still allow for physician-approved participation. If the preparticipation physical notes any respiratory problems, you should contact the athlete's physician for care instructions prior to the athlete's participation.

Asthma occurs in episodes, which means that the condition is always present but becomes a problem only at certain times. Many factors can cause an asthma attack, but in most cases it is brought on by exposure to an allergen, strenuous exercise, or emotional stress. In addition, environmental factors, especially cold environments such as ice rinks, contribute to asthma attacks. It may be wise to counsel asthma sufferers against participation in sports requiring such temperature extremes.

During an attack, small passages in the airway will close down due to muscle contractions and the excessive production of mucus. The force of the person's inspiration will open the airway, allowing air to enter the lungs; however, the expiration will not be as forceful, thus causing the stale air to be trapped and requiring the person to force his or her expirations to move air from the lungs. The air being forced out will produce the wheezing sounds that are heard during an asthma attack.

You must consider the possibility of an asthma attack when you observe labored breathing, which is usually associated with wheezing sounds. The most difficult part of breathing will be expiring. The pulse rate becomes rapid, typically exceeding 120 beats per minute. There should be no chest pains in most cases. You can expect the athlete to become anxious and perhaps appear to be very frightened.

The athlete suffering an asthma attack will sometimes hunch at the shoulders and pull up on the chest in an effort to assist each breath. The athlete may or may not display a blue or grey discoloration of the skin, lips, or nail beds.

To provide care for the athlete having an asthma attack, you should proceed in this manner:

1. Place the athlete in a position that allows for the greatest ease in breathing. This position is usually sitting upright.
2. Reassure the athlete. It is essential that the athlete remain calm.
3. If the athlete is under the care of a physician, follow the physician's directions. If this is not the case or if the athlete does not recover from the episode quickly, have someone alert the EMS system. You cannot predict how the attack will progress or if a more severe attack will follow.
4. Loosen restrictive clothing or equipment.
5. Monitor pulse, respirations, and skin color.
6. Keep the athlete warm, but do not allow overheating to occur.

7. Keep the athlete at rest and help him or her to move into more comfortable positions.

In the case of asthma, the athlete may have prescribed medications that he or she takes for attacks. Unless there are specific regulations that are part of your job description that prevent you from doing so, *assist* the athlete in taking his or her medication. Do *not* attempt to administer medications to the athlete, especially if he or she suffers a loss of consciousness. Your role is to assist by having someone bring the medications, to count out the prescribed dose, and to provide water for taking the pills.

WARNING:

Some asthma victims may develop a severe, prolonged attack or have an attack that does not respond to their medication. Breathing efforts will become very labored, and the chest may distend. The pulse will become very rapid. Very little air will be exchanged, and wheezing will not be heard or will disappear as the severity of the attack increases. An EMS response is critical. Stay with the athlete and be prepared to provide rescue breathing or CPR. Mouth-to-mouth resuscitation may not be successful due to airway obstruction.

SEIZURES

Brain activities can be disturbed by various illnesses and injuries. One result of this disturbance may be irregular electrical activity that can change muscle contractions from smooth movements to uncontrolled contractions. A sudden, uncontrolled contraction is called a *seizure*. Other forms of seizure occur without these contractions being present.

The majority of seizures seen by the coach are due to *epilepsy*. You will be aware of most of your athletes who suffer from this problem from your notes on their preseason physical forms; however, some individuals are unaware that they are epileptic. Unless they have ex-

perienced certain problems, their conditions will not be detected during a preparticipation physical.

Epilepsy sometimes can be attributed to scar tissue or changes in patterns of circulation due to injury or illness; however, the cause of the problems suffered by most victims is unknown. What is known is that epilepsy is an organic problem, not a "mental" disorder. The disease is considered to be chronic, and attacks tend to occur periodically. The athlete who has a known case of epilepsy will be someone who has received a physician's permission to participate and is able to control the episodes with medication. Such an athlete sometimes may not take the prescribed medication or the dose of the medication may no longer be suitable for the athlete. In either case, an episode may occur that requires the coach to provide emergency care.

There are two forms of seizure that may occur as a result of epilepsy. The first is the minor form, called a *petit mal* seizure, and often is not noticeable while it occurs. This form of seizure does not produce convulsions. The athlete suffering such problems will be taking medications that allow for normal activity. If such an athlete suffers a seizure and reports it, you must rest the athlete and contact the attending physician to see what course of action should be taken (e.g., take medication, increase the dose, continue with rest, see the physician, or be transported to a medical facility).

When an epileptic seizure causes convulsions, it is called a *grand mal* seizure. Before the onset of the seizure occurs, the person will often report seeing a bright light, seeing a sudden burst of colors, and/or the sensation of certain odors. There will probably be time for the person to inform you or another athlete that a major seizure is about to occur. The rest of the attack follows the pattern of a convulsive seizure as described below. The care provided should be the same as for any convulsive seizure (see p. 156).

Seizures may be set off by a number of causes other than epilepsy, including head injuries, infection (associated with many of the childhood diseases), high fever, and crises with diabetes management. Many of these seizures will be convulsive ones, with the person typically experiencing a loss of consciousness.

A convulsive seizure will have three phases. During the first phase, consciousness is lost.

The person's body will become rigid, breathing may stop, and there may be a loss of bowel and bladder control. This phase usually lasts no more than 30 seconds. The second phase is the one in which the convulsions take place. In most cases, this phase lasts for no more than 1-2 minutes. The seizure victim may drool and his or her lips may turn blue (cyanosis). Once the convulsions stop, the third phase begins, during which time the person usually regains consciousness and is very confused and drowsy. The most common complaint is a headache.

To provide care for an athlete who is having a convulsive seizure, you should take these steps:

1. Place the athlete on the ground or floor.
2. If it is possible to do so without holding the athlete, loosen any restrictive clothing or equipment. This is often difficult to do.
3. Do what you can to protect the athlete physically during the convulsions (see Figure 14.3). This is done by moving objects out of the way of the athlete or by padding nearby objects. Do *not* try to hold the athlete still during the convulsions.
4. Once the convulsions have stopped, keep the athlete at rest and
   • position the head for drainage from the mouth,

   • reduce his or her embarrassment by having onlookers leave to ensure privacy, and
   • monitor both pulse and breathing.

It is very important that the EMS system be alerted for all cases of convulsive seizure even when the victim is known to suffer from epilepsy as more seizures may follow. In some cases, these seizures may occur without the athlete regaining consciousness. In that instance, you will be dealing with a life-threatening emergency. The sooner the EMS system's personnel are on hand, the safer it will be for the athlete. Remember, you cannot diagnose, nor can you predict what events will follow. Seek professional help by activating the EMS system.

Old guidelines for the care of a person having convulsions called for placing a "bite stick" in the victim's mouth during the seizure. Groups that have studied the prehospital care of convulsing patients no longer recommend the use of these devices because of the dangers involved in placing any object into the mouth of the victim. The object may be broken and swallowed, perhaps obstructing the airway. Seldom does a person bite his or her tongue during a seizure. If local guidelines call for you to use a bite stick, it is recommended that you use a commercial bite stick and not one made by taping together tongue blades.

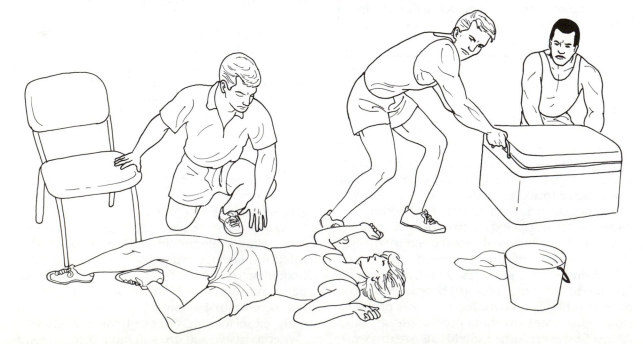

Figure 14.3.   Do what you can to protect athletes experiencing convulsions.

DIABETIC EMERGENCIES

Many individuals who have diabetes wear medical alert bracelets or necklaces or carry an information card. These items can be of assistance if you do not know the person who is having the emergency. Some individuals having a diabetic emergency may act as if they are intoxicated on alcohol. Never assume that the problem is due simply to alcohol until you are able to rule out diabetes, high fever, head injury, stroke, and drug abuse.

The person who suffers from diabetes has a problem with taking sugar (specifically, glucose) from the bloodstream into the cells. This process requires that there be a proper balance of sugar and insulin available. If there is not enough insulin, the sugar in circulation cannot be used.

Insulin-dependent (type I) diabetes occurs in people who cannot produce and secrete insulin. Although this disorder's onset can begin in a person's 20s, it is typically a problem of childhood and has been called "juvenile diabetes." Noninsulin-dependent diabetes (type II) occurs when the individual cannot produce or utilize the needed level of insulin. Since this is a problem associated with adults, it has been called "maturity-onset diabetes."

Many cases of diabetes can go undetected for years. The problem, when discovered, can be controlled by a physician-approved diet or by diet and doses of insulin. If you have an athlete who is using insulin, an emergency may develop if he or she uses too little or too much insulin for his or her diet and activity levels.

If too little insulin is available, either as a result of missing a dose, using a dose that is too low for the activity level, or overeating, then too much sugar will be in the blood. This is known as *hyperglycemia*. If left untreated, the problem can become a life-threatening *diabetic coma*. The athlete who is developing a diabetic coma will have any or all of the following symptoms and signs:

- A dry mouth and thirst
- Pain in the abdomen (possible vomiting)
- Restlessness
- Confusion

As the problem continues, the following will be noted:

- Confusion developing into a state of stupor or unconsciousness

- Breathing becoming deep (possibly heavy sighing)
- The breath smelling of acetone (the odor of nail-polish remover)
- The pulse becoming rapid and weak
- The skin becoming dry, red, and warm
- The eyes appearing sunken

Problems that lead to diabetic coma have a gradual onset. It will usually take several days for the athlete's condition to become severe. If you are dealing with a possible case of hyperglycemia related to diabetes or if a diabetic coma is probably developing, alert the EMS system to provide immediate transport. Keep the athlete at rest and treat for shock.

When a diabetic takes too much insulin, does not eat properly to provide the needed level of sugar, or has overexerted him- or herself, the sugar level will be lower than that needed by the brain. This condition is *hypoglycemia*, or too little sugar in the blood. In a diabetic, this can develop into *insulin shock*, which may lead to brain damage or death.

Insulin shock, unlike diabetic coma, has a rapid onset, with symptoms and signs developing in a matter of minutes. The diabetic athlete who is developing insulin shock will have the following symptoms and signs:

- Intense hunger
- Rapid, full pulse
- Dizziness and/or headache
- Pale skin that will be cold and clammy (due to profuse sweating)
- Increased saliva production (possibly drooling)
- Changes in behavior, perhaps becoming hostile or aggressive
- Possible fainting or unconsciousness
- Possible convulsions

To provide care for the alert athlete who may be developing insulin shock, you should take the following steps:

1. Have someone alert the EMS system.
2. Provide sugar in the form of orange juice, granular sugar, candy, or a sweetened soft drink. Make certain that the source contains sugar and not an artificial sweetener. You may want to keep a roll of lifesavers or a candy bar in your first aid kit.
3. Treat for shock and position the head for drainage.
4. Monitor pulse and breathing.

If the athlete is unconscious, do what is directed above, but do not administer anything orally. Some states' guidelines for emergency care may allow you to sprinkle granulated sugar under the athlete's tongue. If this is allowed in your locality, sprinkle only a few crystals at a time from your fingers, not from the pack. Your medical or legal advisor will be able to tell you if this is allowed in your state for your level of training. The danger of inducing vomiting is the major reason why most localities do not allow these actions.

Whenever the athlete is conscious and has suffered a diabetic emergency and you cannot tell whether the problem is developing into a diabetic coma or insulin shock, give the athlete sugar. You will not be harming the athlete in a diabetic coma, and you may save a life if his or her problem is insulin shock.

ACUTE ABDOMEN

As noted in the sections on injuries, abdominal pain can be spread over a large area or can occur away from the site of injury. Although certain problems tend to present specific pain patterns, there are many cases in which this is not true. Never assume that a medical problem that produces pain in the abdomen is minor. Always find out whether the problem may be due to injury. Some abdominal injuries, including bruised organs associated with contact sports and gymnastics, do not produce significant pain for several days.

Many medical problems can produce abdominal pain and distress. The nature of the difficulties can be as minor as simple indigestion or as major as a perforated ulcer or an inflamed body organ. The female athlete's problem may include those associated with menstruation, reproductive organ inflammation, ovarian cysts, and pregnancy (including an implantation outside the uterus, or ectopic pregnancy). With so many problems possible, many of which can become serious or life threatening in a short period of time, the coach is well advised to consider all abdominal complaints carefully.

Consider the athlete who has abdominal complaints to be having a problem serious enough to require response by the EMS or other health care professionals if any of the following occurs:

- Sustained abdominal pain confined to one area or widespread
- Fainting or loss of consciousness
- Nausea with or without vomiting
- A rapid pulse and/or rapid shallow breathing (usually associated with the pain)
- Apparent fever
- Profuse sweating
- Diarrhea or constipation (at the time of the problem or within the last few days)
- A tender abdomen, involving one area or the entire abdomen
- An unusually soft or rigid abdomen
- Distention or swelling of the abdomen
- Muscle spasms of the abdominal wall
- Reports of bleeding from the rectum, blood in the urine, or nonmenstrual bleeding from the vagina
- Any unusual premenstrual or menstrual problems
- Guarding of the abdomen, where the athlete tries to lie perfectly still or pulls the knees up to the chest
- The presence of any other symptoms, signs, or conditions such as previous injury, infection, respiratory or heart problems, diabetes, and so on.

When faced with such problems, have someone alert the EMS system while you keep the athlete at rest. When required, ensure an open airway. Place the athlete on his or her back and flex the knees to reduce strain on the abdominal muscles. Stay alert for vomiting and monitor pulse and breathing. Cover the athlete, but do not allow overheating to take place. Administer nothing orally. Because the athlete's condition may worsen without warning, use the basic assessment interview techniques (see chapter 3) to obtain information concerning the type of pain, when it started, any unusual bowel or bladder problems, recent bleeding, what liquids the athlete may have consumed, and the nature of the last meal and when it was eaten.

Be certain that you and the athlete follow all recommendations from the attending physician when an athlete who has had abdominal problems returns to activity. Never allow the athlete to participate if any of the indications of abdominal distress are present. Participation should be delayed or strictly limited for those athletes who have had recent problems with vomiting or diarrhea. Dehydration can become a serious problem as it develops quickly.

INFECTIOUS DISEASES

Consider the possibility of an infectious disease whenever you detect, or the athlete reports, fever, profuse sweating, vomiting, diarrhea, constipation, pain (stiff neck, headache, earache, sore throat, chest or abdominal pain), lesions of the skin or skin rashes, coughing, or sneezing. In such cases, rest the athlete and be certain that he or she sees a physician. If you note that the athlete is "very sick" by a layperson's standards or if you note a rapid, obvious decline in the athlete's condition, call for an EMS response.

Infection can be spread by direct contact with the infected person (even the simple act of shaking hands may pass on the agents responsible for many infections), direct contact with infected body fluids, contact with droplets (including the microscopic droplets that are coughed or sneezed into the air), and indirect contact (such as grasping a doorknob previously touched by an infected person who has droplets on the hand). It is obvious that the infected athlete who is capable of passing on the infection should be isolated from others. Unfortunately, many diseases are in a contagious state before a person is aware of his or her own infection (e.g., influenza).

When appropriate, you should keep the athlete who has an infectious disease away from others and from equipment or commonly shared items that may become contaminated. Mats, apparatus surfaces, shared equipment, water bottles and cups, and locker and shower room surfaces may become contaminated. In fact, contact with the same environmental surfaces may be the way that disease is transmitted to others. This is particularly true if the infection can be spread from the skin (e.g., athlete's foot) or by secretions or blood from open cuts and lesions (e.g., infectious hepatitis). Whenever you are dealing with the potential of disease transmission, follow the recommendations of the attending physician.

Certain diseases may require limiting activity to protect other athletes. An example would be some open skin lesions or skin infections. The athlete may not be allowed to participate in wrestling where direct contact with a person or with the mat may transmit the disease. The same is true in gymnastics, where contact with apparatus and mats provide the opportunity for disease transmission. Again, the attending physician can inform you of the dangers of transmission.

Certain skin problems that should be evaluated by a health care professional are often treated by coaches. In most cases, no harm is done; however, some serious problems can be overlooked. There is always a potential danger in recommending treatments for apparently simple problems such as "jock itch" (jock rash). Because you cannot make a diagnosis and because the symptoms reported by the athlete may not be complete, a different problem may exist. The source of infection could be an organism that can not be limited by the medication you recommend. The problem could be due to crab lice that could infest other people. Perhaps the athlete has herpes and needs special attention. Your recommendations for treating jock itch could delay proper care and may allow the athlete to transmit the infection. Be sure that any athlete who has a skin problem or infection is evaluated by a physician or an appropriate health care professional (e.g., school nurse) who can determine if additional care is needed.

Fungal infections of the groin (jock itch) and athlete's foot in its early stages usually respond well to keeping the problem areas dry, wearing clean clothing, and using fungicide medications. Once beyond the stage of simple itching, or if early treatment fails, the athlete must consult a physician. Remember that skin infections that are treated without the benefit of a physician's diagnosis and care tend to recur more frequently than do those that are treated by a physician.

SUBSTANCE ABUSE

It is sad to say that substance abuse by athletes is a problem, and it is even more alarming when one notes that it is on the increase. Many experts predict that this will be the trend for some time to come.

Whenever alcohol or drug abuse is detected, the athlete should be given the appropriate professional medical care and counseling. The role of the coach is one of guiding the athlete to the proper source of care and support and is not one of total crisis intervention and management. An athlete with substance-abuse problems has as great a need for advanced care as one who suffers a bone fracture.

At one time, simple guidelines were prepared to allow coaches to detect the abuse of alcohol or specific classes of drugs. Today, many substance abusers mix drugs and alcohol or use several classes of drugs in combination. The signs produced by such actions can be very confusing even for allied health and medical personnel. What follows are some general guidelines in terms of detecting abuse, evaluating the need for emergency action, and providing emergency care.

Alcohol Abuse

Look for the typical signs of excessive alcohol use, including the odor of alcohol on the breath or clothing, unsteadiness or emphasis of movement, slurred speech or the failure to carry on normal conversation, a flushed appearance, profuse sweating, nausea, and vomiting. Withdrawal from alcohol may show itself by the person becoming restless and displaying atypical behavior. In advanced cases, the person may have hallucinations, shaking hands (gross tremor), and possibly convulsions.

Stimulants (Uppers)

The person abusing stimulants will probably show excitement, an increased pulse rate, and rapid speech. Higher levels of abuse tend to show these signs as well as dilated pupils, a dry mouth, loss of appetite, and loss of sleep. The individual tends to become more apprehensive and is often uncooperative.

Depressants (Downers)

The person abusing depressants will probably show a loss of some body coordination. In addition to this, there may be a "sleepiness" or "sluggishness" noticed. Speech will be slowed or the individual will lack the coordination for normal conversation. Both pulse and breathing rates will be slowed.

Anabolic Steroids

The use of anabolic steroids to gain muscle bulk and increase strength has no ethical place in sports at any level of competition. This class of drugs has been outlawed by most national governing bodies for Olympic sports and by the International Olympic Committee.

The popularity of anabolic steroids has increased dramatically over the last decade to the point where elite athletes believe they cannot compete fairly without the aid of the drug. Unfortunately, now even high school athletes are experimenting with anabolic steroids in the hope of bulking up.

At present, scientific studies have yet to prove that anabolic steroids taken in megadoses provide either a strength or an aerobic advantage. What is well documented, however, is that anabolic steroids have many side effects, some of which are reversible once the individual stops taking the drug. Some of the side effects can precipitate life-threatening conditions.

Anabolic steroids cause an increase in protein production in the body. They are closely related to the androgenic (male) hormone testosterone, which is responsible for the increased muscle mass in males during the adolescent growth spurt. Athletes who take anabolic steroids exhibit certain physical and behavioral characteristics that can alert the informed coach of possible abuse. Among the readily discernible physical changes in an abuser are these signs:

- Flare-up of acne and increased oiliness of the skin
- Loss of hair (general thinning or localized baldness)
- Sudden weight gain (10 to 20 pounds in 6 to 12 weeks)
- Nosebleeds
- Enlargement of breast tissue (male athlete)
- Atrophy of the testicles (male athlete)

Because anabolic steroids are closely related chemically to testosterone, these drugs have a masculinizing effect on female athletes. Such physical changes are *not* reversible. The masculine characteristics observed in the female include the following:

- Deepening of the voice
- Abnormal growth of hair on the face and body
- Development of muscle bulk similar to that seen in male athletes
- Impaired reproductive capacity and menstrual cycle changes ranging from early onset to scanty or absent menses

- Enlargement of the clitoris
- Reduction in breast tissue

Major medical problems precipitated by large doses of anabolic steroids include cardiovascular complications such as early hardening of the arteries, sterility, diabetes, and liver abnormalities, including cancer.

WARNING:

If the athlete using anabolic steroids has not completed his or her adolescent growth spurt, the drug may cause premature closure of the epiphyses, thus stunting growth.

Behaviorally the athlete on steroids shows an increase in aggression, which may not be noticed in athletic events where some aggression is part of the game. However, in interpersonal relationships, the increased aggression is easily noted, even during the turbulent teens. The athlete will also have more frequent and more intense mood changes than is typical of adolescents.

As with all drugs, the best advice concerning anabolic steroids is to stay away. The dangers outweigh the somewhat-suspect benefits.

Narcotics

These are typically drugs that are derived from opium or manufactured synthetically and are noted for altering the user's sensibility or inducing a state of stupor. The person's vital signs—pulse rate, breathing rate, and skin temperature—will all be below normal. The pupils will usually be constricted. The person will typically become sleepy and not want to do even the simplest of acts. The muscles will be very relaxed. Most cases will display an increase in sweating (often profuse).

Hallucinogens (Mind-Altering Drugs)

The person's pulse rate quickens and the breathing rate may rise. The pupils will usually be dilated. At a certain level of abuse, the face may appear flushed. The concept of real time

is usually lost and so is an awareness of the true environment. The person may hallucinate (seeing or hearing things that are not present or distorting the perception of the environment). What the person says to you will often make no sense. The mind-altering drug user may become aggressive, sometimes without warning.

Mind-Alerting Drugs (Nonhallucinogenic)

These include cannabis products such as marijuana, "hash" (hashish), and THC. The body's reactions often depend on the strength of the compounds used and previous exposure to the drug. As the effects of the drug increase, the user will experience euphoria and a relaxing of inhibitions. Some users will have an increase in appetite. Intoxication and its associated disorientation occur long before overdose. Once overdose is reached, fatigue will occur. Changes in typical behavior develop, including paranoia. In some cases, psychoses have been reported.

Volatile Chemicals

These substances include compounds that are found in spray paints, glues, cleaning fluids, and polishes. The person will usually appear dazed and will sometimes show a detachment from reality. The membranes of the nose and mouth may appear swollen. The person may complain of numbness or tingling in the head. In some cases, paint or other foreign substances may be detected around the nose and mouth.

Drug Withdrawal

The effects of withdrawing from habitual drug abuse can vary greatly according to the level of dependency, the substance(s) abused, and the tolerance of the individual to withdrawal. Look for anxiety or extreme restlessness, a high level of irritability, shaking, nausea, profuse sweating, and increased breathing and pulse rates.

If you discover that an athlete is abusing or withdrawing from a substance, consider this situation to be an emergency. You cannot tell how the person will act or how his or her condition may develop. When possible, interview the victim as well as others who may have relevant information. Begin by using the term *medications* rather than drugs. Many people will worry about the legal problems of drug abuse to the point that they let themselves or another person suffer a medical emergency rather than supply information. If the answers you receive do not make sense or are too general to be useful, switch to the term *drugs* when asking questions. Do not depend too greatly on the information supplied by the abuse or withdrawal victim or by others in terms of what may have been abused or how much of the drug was consumed.

Make certain that you and others at the scene are safe from harm. Call for an EMS response. In some areas, you can call the poison-control center or drug-abuse center to receive directions for care. Otherwise, keep the person at rest, ensure an open airway, and stay alert for vomiting. Treat for shock and attempt to reassure the drug-abuse or withdrawal victim.

WARNING:

If the drug in question is suspected to be PCP, make certain that you and others are safe and that the EMS system is aware of this information. The PCP user often has lost the concept of right and wrong and is subject to becoming violent. If you do not stay alert, you may be harmed or even killed by the abuser.

As you assess the emergency situation, never assume that drugs have been abused or that drug abuse is the only cause of the problem. Remember that diabetic emergencies, head injuries, stroke, and severe respiratory problems may produce signs similar to drug abuse. Remember also that a person who has abused drugs may also have injured him- or herself. Be sure to check for additional injury.

SUMMARY AND RECOMMENDATIONS

A variety of possible medical problems and emergencies may have to be detected by the coach. This requires you to use the information provided in the preseason physical exam and carefully apply your assessment skills.

Keep the following points in mind:

1. As a coach, you must stay alert to detect and care for problems involving chest or abdominal pains, difficult breathing, seizures, diabetic emergencies, infectious illnesses, and substance abuse.

2. In most cases, the problems you face will be related to known problems. You will have to be aware of which athletes have particular health problems and what their physicians expect you to do in case of a medical emergency.

3. Many athletes will be encouraged to participate even though they have a medical problem. Asthma is a good example. Most asthma victims having an attack will have indications of respiratory distress and produce a wheezing sound on expiration. The care for the problem is essentially the same as for respiratory distress. In localities where it is allowed, you may help the alert asthma victim to take prescribed medications.

4. Substance abuse may go undetected by the athlete's physician or may start after the season begins. Once detected, you must not ignore the situation. Have the athlete receive professional substance-abuse counseling and care. If a medical emergency occurs due to substance abuse or withdrawal, alert the EMS system, provide emotional support, ensure an open airway, be prepared for vomiting, and treat for shock. Monitor pulse and respirations. Make certain that you have ruled out other medical problems and injuries as the cause of the problem.

Chapter 15
Moving the Injured Athlete

Effective educational programs have reduced the great pressures that were once placed on a coach to move an injured athlete quickly from the playing field or away from a piece of apparatus. Today, most coaches, fans, and athletes understand the importance of assessing the injuries and providing certain elements of care before the athlete is moved. If you experience the rare situation in which people ask you to move an athlete prematurely for the sake of a time schedule, ignore the request and give the first consideration to the athlete.

Likewise, you must discourage your athletes from attempting to remove themselves from the playing field when they are injured and ignore requests for them to do so. Help them to understand that it is wrong to try to limp or crawl from where they were injured. Such actions might lead to additional injury that could mean a prolonged period of rehabilitation, being unable to participate in the sport again, or a serious lifelong problem.

THE DECISION TO MOVE AN ATHLETE

The injured athlete should not be moved unless *all* the following conditions are met:

- The primary survey is complete, and the athlete is breathing adequately and has an adequate pulse.
- All major and moderate bleeding are controlled.
- There are no indications of developing shock, and breathing and pulse rates are within the acceptable range.
- The appropriate aspects of the secondary survey are complete, and there is no indication of neck or spinal injury.

- The athlete is conscious.
- There are no indications of serious head injury.
- The mechanism of injury does not indicate the clear possibility of serious head, neck, back, or internal injuries.
- All possible fractures are splinted or properly immobilized.

Unless *all* the above are found to be true, care must be rendered where the athlete lies. An EMS response must be requested to allow emergency care professionals to provide the necessary care before moving any athlete who may have respiratory or cardiac arrest, uncontrollable bleeding, developing shock or unstable vital signs, possible neck or spinal injuries, serious head injury, or altered states of awareness.

This does not mean that you cannot reposition the athlete as dictated by care, for example, to provide CPR, to reposition a limb for adequate splinting (if properly trained), or to move one athlete off of another so that the second athlete can receive basic life support measures. It does mean that all activity around the injured athlete must come to a stop and the rules of basic emergency care must be followed. Moving the athlete too soon simply to speed up play is unacceptable.

HOW TO MOVE THE INJURED ATHLETE

The techniques used to move or reposition an injured person are called *moves*. Some of these moves can be performed by one trained individual, while others require the help of additional trained persons. Before the sporting event begins, make certain that there are enough trained people at the contest, or enough adults who are willing to help and follow your directions to allow you to move an injured athlete if the need arises. Athletes may be used if they volunteer to help and you believe them to be capable of assisting. Do not depend on the help of other athletes if you consider them too young to be given the responsibility of assisting with a move. No athlete should be "ordered" to help with a move. The decision to assume that responsibility should be the athlete's.

You and anyone who assists with a move *must* use correct lifting techniques to avoid lower-back and knee injury and to ensure proper balance throughout the move. Anyone moving the athlete should take these precautions:

- Be familiar with the move to be used.
- Think through the move before attempting it. If the person "sees" any difficulties, he or she should request help.
- Do not attempt to move, lift, or assist the injured athlete unless the person is certain that he or she can control the weight involved.
- Establish firm footing before initiating the move, and be certain of footing and balance throughout the move.
- Begin the move from a balanced position, and remain strongly aware of balance throughout the move.
- Remain aware of proper breathing to avoid holding the breath during the move.

- Protect the back by lifting with the legs. The person must bend at the knees when required to do so, positioning one foot slightly behind the other, and keeping the back straight during a lift.
- Keep the back straight when carrying the injured athlete.

The Rescuer Assist

In most cases, the injured athlete will be able to walk alone or with the help of one or two persons. It is best to assist this athlete even if it does not appear that help is needed. Do *not* risk the chance of additional injury by assuming that the athlete will be able to help him- or herself or that the condition of the athlete will not change.

The one-rescuer assist requires you to take the following steps:

1. Stand beside the athlete and place the arm that is closest to you around your neck. Keep a hold on the athlete's wrist. If the athlete has an upper-extremity injury, stand on the uninjured side. If the lower extremity has been injured, the athlete will find it easier to maintain his or her balance if you stand on the injured side.
2. Place your free arm around the athlete's waist.
3. Walk with the athlete, making any necessary adjustments for balance. Do not force the speed of the move but adjust

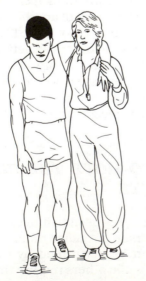 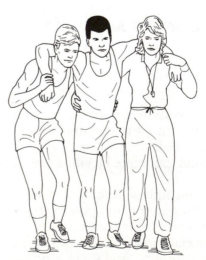

Figure 15.1. The one- and two-rescuer assists.

to the speed of the athlete. If necessary, request the athlete to slow down if the pace is too fast.

This same move can be carried out with one person on each side of the athlete (two-rescuer assist). When the move is in progress, the two people moving the athlete should walk out of step (avoid walking that will have them both using the same foot on a given step, i.e., marching). This is done to avoid causing the athlete to sway with the persons as they walk. Both the one- and the two-rescuer assists are illustrated in Figure 15.1

The Extremity Lift

The extremity lift is a simple move that requires two persons to lift and carry the injured athlete. It is such an easy move that it often is selected when it should not be used. This move must never be attempted if there is *any* possibility of serious injuries to the head, neck, spine, shoulders, pelvis, hips, or knees. All possible fractures of the upper and lower extremities *must be splinted*. (See Figure 15.2):

1. Begin with the athlete placed on his or her back.
2. Have the athlete flex the knees.

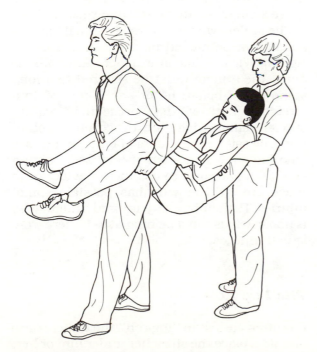

Figure 15.2. The extremity lift.

3. One person should kneel at the athlete's head and place the hands under the athlete's shoulders.
4. The second person should stand at the athlete's feet and lean forward and grasp the athlete's wrists.
5. The person at the athlete's head should tell the other person to pull the athlete into a sitting position. This pulling should not be done if there are any signs of injuries of the shoulders or upper limbs. Instead, the "head" person pushes the athlete into position.
6. The "head" person should reach under the athlete's armpits and grasp the wrists.
7. The "foot" person should turn his or her back to the athlete, kneel down, and grasp the athlete's legs behind the knees.
8. The "head" person should direct the lift and move so that both persons will lift, carry, stop, and place the athlete down as a unit. They should walk out of step to keep from swinging the athlete.

The Two- and Four-Handed Seat Carries

Two people are required for a two-handed seat carry, while three persons are necessary to complete a four-handed seat carry. The injured athlete must be able to cooperate with the people doing the carry.

The two-handed seat carry requires the two people doing the carry to grasp wrists as shown in Figure 15.3. They keep their other hands free to provide back support for the athlete. The athlete sits or is placed onto the seat formed by the persons' hands and is lifted and carried. Both persons should walk out of step to avoid swinging the athlete.

The four-handed seat requires the persons to grasp the wrists as shown in Figure 15.4. The athlete sits or is placed on this seat, and the same principles are used to lift and carry the athlete that were used for the two-handed seat. Because the two persons doing the carry cannot provide support for the athlete's back, a third person *must* follow in case such support is needed. The athlete should also be encouraged to put his or her arms around the shoulders and neck of the carriers.

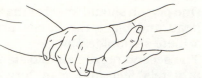

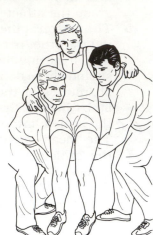

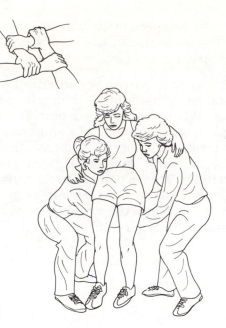

Figure 15.4. Performing the four-handed seat carry.

MOVING TO A STRETCHER

There are times when it is best to place the injured athlete on a stretcher before moving him or her to another location to complete care. The availability of a stretcher does not mean that it should be used for every case in which an athlete is unable to walk off the playing surface. The basic rules of when not to move an injured athlete still apply (see p. 168).

The athlete who has possible spinal injuries should not be moved until an extrication or rigid cervical collar is in place. After this is done, the athlete must be secured to a long spine board before he or she is moved to a stretcher. Both of these procedures require special training; therefore, the coach and other nonprofessional providers of emergency care who have not had such specialized training should not attempt to use these devices or to move any athlete who has possible spinal injuries. Remember, any injured athlete who is unconscious *must* be treated as if there were spinal injuries.

The Log Roll

It is often easiest to "log roll" the athlete onto one side, place the stretcher under him or her, and gently lower him or her back onto the

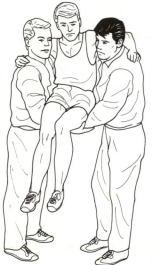

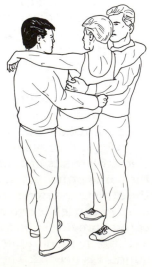

Figure 15.3. Performing the two-handed seat carry.

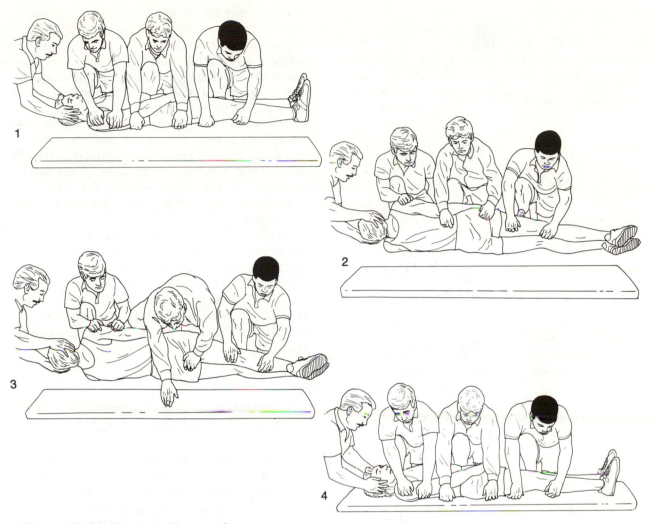

Figure 15.5. The log roll using four rescuers.

stretcher (see Figure 15.5). It is recommended that four people be used in performing the log roll as this will enable you to move the athlete's body as a unit, thus avoiding any twists of the head and trunk or the undesired repositioning of the limbs.

The Direct Ground Lift

If the athlete is to be lifted onto a stretcher (always necessary if you are using a wheeled stretcher), you should use at least two helpers and do the following:

1. Place the stretcher at the athlete's head or feet and at a right angle to the body (so you will not trip over it).
2. Kneel at the athlete's head and place one hand under the neck and the other hand under the upper back.

3. The first helper should kneel at the athlete's waist and place one arm under the waist and the other arm under the hips.
4. The second helper should kneel at the athlete's lower legs and place one arm under the knees and the other arm under the ankles.
5. Direct everyone to lift the athlete to their knees.

At this point, the actions taken depend on how you can position the stretcher. For example, if the stretcher can be placed directly in front of you and your helpers (see Figure 15.6), then you can direct everyone to roll the athlete to their chests, have the stretcher placed in front of you and your helpers, and then direct everyone to lower and place the athlete slowly, face up, onto the stretcher.

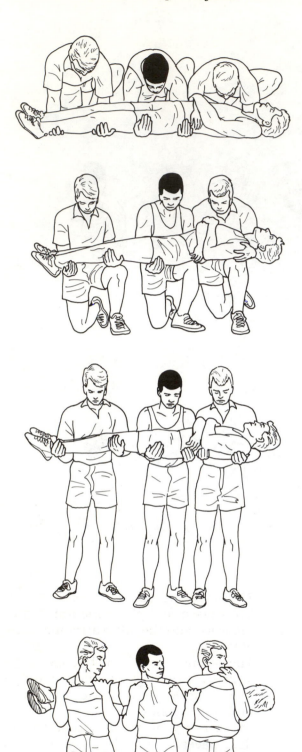

Figure 15.6. The direct ground lift.

There may be situations in which it is necessary to move an athlete who is lying against something that will obstruct any attempt to move the stretcher in front of you. You may also experience the problem of not having anyone available to place the stretcher once the athlete has been lifted. In either case, direct everyone to move to a standing position, roll the athlete to their chests, and walk toward the stretcher. Remind all those involved in the lift to use their legs, not their backs, in lifting the athlete. The procedure to lower the athlete as a unit onto the stretcher is simply the reverse of the lift.

Once the athlete is placed on the stretcher, make certain that he or she is secured to the stretcher by belts or straps before being wheeled or carried. *Never* move someone on a stretcher unless the person is properly secured. In addition, when carrying a stretcher, everyone should walk out of step to avoid any swinging motions.

SUMMARY AND RECOMMENDATIONS

The coach must take great care in moving an injured athlete. The decision to move or to wait until more highly trained help arrives is critical. The results of the primary and the secondary assessments will determine whether the athlete can be moved.

Keep the following points in mind:

1. There are some absolutes in terms of moving an injured athlete. Do *not* move an athlete who has respiratory or cardiac arrest, uncontrolled moderate or serious bleeding, developing shock or unacceptable pulse and/or breathing rates, possible neck or spinal injuries, possible head injuries, possible internal injuries, unsplinted fractures or who is unconscious or has altered states of awareness. Instead, provide the necessary initial care and make certain that an EMS system response has been requested.

2. The techniques used to reposition or move an injured athlete are called moves.

3. The one-rescuer assist can be used to help the injured athlete walk.

4. The extremity lift can be used by two persons to lift and carry the athlete by the shoulders and knees.
5. Seat carries can be performed by two or three persons.
6. An injured athlete can be moved to a stretcher by way of a log roll or the direct ground lift.
7. Anyone placed on a stretcher must be properly secured before being moved.

PART III
Follow-Up Care

Chapter 16
Principles of Rehabilitation

The rehabilitation of the injured athlete usually requires limited participation by the coach. A physician will decide what is to be done, when and how it will be done, and when the athlete is ready for participation. Most programs will be planned by the physician, certified athletic trainer, and/or a physical therapist, with much of the activity being done away from the school or organization that sponsors the sporting event. However, you may be asked to supervise an athlete's rehabilitation program, so it is essential that you understand the basics of rehabilitation.

As a coach, you should not attempt to design and carry out your own rehabilitation programs. Likewise, you should not offer to supervise any aspect of a rehabilitation program for which you do not have the needed training and experience to conduct the activity safely. The materials presented in the remainder of this book will introduce you to the principles of rehabilitation and serve as a guide to help you carry out any duties assigned by the attending physician.

FOLLOW-UP CARE

Following any trauma to an athlete's body, there is localized tissue damage that requires time for repair and healing. Rest is essential to keep stress on the injured part to a minimum. However, when joints and muscles are injured, rest and time may not be enough to guarantee the athlete's complete recovery. The stress of the sport activity may be too great even for the newly healed injury. Unfortunately, this can mean reinjury and additional delays in the healing process.

As an example, consider the case of an athlete who has sprained an ankle. On returning to activity, the athlete has a three-strike count on him or her:

- *Strike One.* A ligament is an inelastic structure. Once this band of tissue is stretched, it remains stretched. This means that the joint has lost some of its stability even with the mildest sprain (the simple stretching of the ligament). The instability may be minimal, but it is enough to affect performance and to give the athlete an uneasy feeling.
- *Strike Two.* Healing takes place by substitution, not by duplication. Any scar tissue that is formed is neither as strong nor as elastic as the tissue it replaces. Muscle injuries are notorious for recurring because the inelastic "plug" of scar tissue that is formed does not stretch like the elastic muscles.
- *Strike Three.* The athlete's level of fitness diminishes with inactivity. It is estimated that an athlete can suffer a loss of 2%-3% of his or her strength for every day of imposed inactivity. An athlete needs strength for the correct execution of skills and as a first line of defense against injury and reinjury.

What can the coach do? You must ensure that the athlete is placed in a program that will fill the gap between healing and full recovery. This program is rehabilitation—the restoring of the injured part to the level of function required for the athlete's particular activity. To do this, the rehabilitation program must fulfill three functions:

- Compensate for any loss of joint stability by strengthening the muscles, known as secondary stabilizers, that cross a joint and control its movements.

- Regain the strength and flexibility of any injured muscle tissue.
- Help the athlete to regain the level of fitness that diminished as a result of inactivity. In fact, the athlete should be in *better* shape on returning.

When to Start

Rehabilitation of an injury should begin as soon as possible but *only* after the attending physician has given you written permission to do so. Any athlete who has a serious injury should be examined, treated, and assigned to an appropriate rehabilitation program by a physician. Generally, the athlete will have to be reevaluated both before the rehabilitation program can begin and before returning to the activity.

Rehabilitation should be delayed if the athlete has pain and swelling. The bottom line in a rehabilitation program can be phrased in this way: If it hurts to do the exercise, or the exercise causes additional swelling, do not do it . . . you are not ready! At the same time, keep in mind the old expression, "no pain, no gain." Of course, the pain being mentioned is that of restorative exertion as the muscles, heart, and lungs are stressed to regain optimum fitness. This pain is different from that experienced when the athlete is doing too much too soon, which is pain that is localized at the injury site and the surrounding areas. Rehabilitation is hard work, but a measure of the effectiveness of this work is *not* additional pain and swelling.

The Role of the Physician

The physician should examine and evaluate the extent of the athlete's injury and then provide the necessary treatment. The athlete will have to be reevaluated both before rehabilitation can begin and before returning to the activity. Any problems experienced during rehabilitation will have to be evaluated by the physician and can lead to delaying or modifying the rehabilitation program.

You should be in contact with the attending physician and receive an outline of the planned rehabilitation program, which should define your role. The physician may wish to delay the start of the program or periodically modify it to better suit the needs of the individual athlete.

Mental Factors

The attitudes taken by you, the athlete, fellow athletes and peers, the attending physician, and the athlete's family and friends will all have an important role in the success of the rehabilitation program. It is essential that you discuss rehabilitation during the first team meeting with your athletes. You must let them know long before the first injury occurs why rehabilitation is so important and how serious you are about the programs. The more serious you are, the more likely the athletes will also be serious.

Next, you should try to establish a relationship with each athlete that will allow you to gain the necessary trust to carry out a rehabilitation program effectively when the athlete is depressed or worried about the length of time he or she will be away from participation. This rapport will be beneficial whether or not the athlete is ever injured. However, the rehabilitation program has a greater chance for success if the athlete believes your judgement is trustworthy and your reassurances sincere.

KEY PHYSICAL FACTORS IN REHABILITATION

The rehabilitation program should be a systematic approach that is designed to return the athlete to his or her preinjury condition. Certain physical factors may become diminished as a direct result of the injury and inactivity. The rehabilitation programs must address these physical factors:

- Normal range of motion or flexibility
- Strength
- Muscular endurance
- Cardiorespiratory (cardiopulmonary) endurance
- Skill (agility and coordination)

Each of these must be regained and developed in the exact order shown above. One physical factor provides the foundation for the next one. Therefore, you should proceed from one stage of rehabilitation to the next as directed by the attending physician.

Range of Motion

Range-of-motion exercises should be initiated as soon as you receive the attending physician's approval. The initial exercises may be limited because of the restricted range of pain-free motion.

The exercises are simple, isolated movement patterns that are used to regain the normal range of motion in the injured joint. Each exercise consists of moving the joint (not forcing it) through one of its normal movement patterns (e.g., pointing the toes). These exercises accomplish two additional goals:

- They decrease congestion in the injured area by stimulating the return of blood to the heart (venous drainage).
- The early motion prevents adhesions from developing between moving tissues.

It is important to avoid forcing the motion as this can aggravate the healing tissues and defeat the purpose of the exercises. If the exercise is carried out too soon or is forced to go beyond the point of discomfort, additional swelling and tissue damage will probably occur. As a result, the range of motion will actually decrease. Sample flexibility exercises are illustrated in Figure 16.1

Strength

Once the range of motion has become nearly normal (as determined by comparison with the uninjured part), you will probably be directed to switch the program's emphasis to strength-gaining exercises. Carefully follow the physician's directions. You must be careful not to start these exercises too early as this will benefit only a limited range within the joint's entire range of motion.

There are three different types of exercise that can be used to build up strength: isometric, isotonic, and isokinetic. Specific examples of each are presented in the ACEP Level 2 Sport

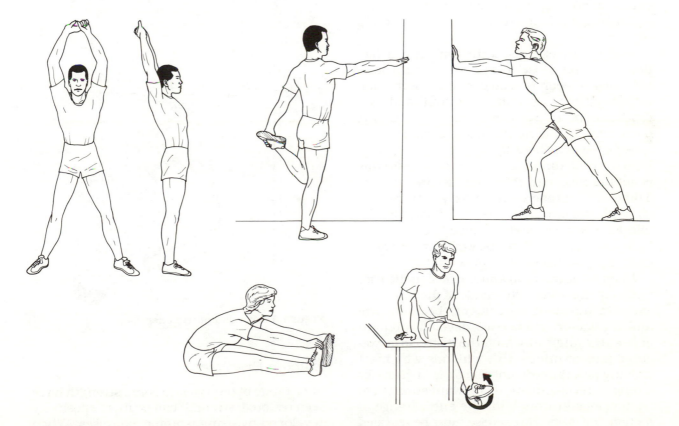

Figure 16.1. Sample exercises for improving range of motion.

Physiology Course described at the beginning of this book.

Isometric Exercises

In an isometric (static contraction) exercise, the muscles contract maximally against opposing muscles or an immovable object, but no movement takes place in the joint. Isometrics are regularly used at the beginning of rehabilitation to help prevent the wasting away (atrophy) of muscles that are not being used as in the case of casted limbs. Such exercises do not irritate the healing tissues.

As an example of this type of exercise, consider what is done in the early phase of knee rehabilitation, when an exercise known as the straight-leg raise is recommended. The injured leg is kept straight as the athlete lies on the back and contracts the front thigh muscles and lifts the straight leg 6-8 inches off the floor. Because there is no movement at the knee except for the sliding of the kneecap upward along the surface of the femur (patellar surface), the exercise is isometric for the knee and isotonic for the hip. If the athlete is suffering from a knee sprain, in most cases the muscles can be exercised regularly by doing straight-leg raises without stressing the recovering tissues.

In isometric exercises, the muscle contraction is always close to the maximum and is held for 4-6 seconds. The period of contraction is followed by relaxation for 1 minute and then repeated one to five times. This approach is used only in a conditioning program where muscle tissue is healthy and is able to generate a near-maximum contraction. Because this is not the case with the rehabilitating athlete, a different approach is necessary. Contraction strength and duration must be adjusted for the tolerance and the level of muscle use of each individual athlete. Examples of isometric exercises are illustrated in Figure 16.2

When some strength and range of motion are restored, the initial advantage of the isometric exercise (no joint movement) becomes the limiting factor. Isometrics develop strength only at the angle at which the exercise is executed plus or minus 15°, which is why most training programs do not rely on isometrics for strength development. If you want strength to be developed throughout the entire range of motion, the isometric exercise must be repeated at different angles. Also, isometric exercises do not build muscular endurance.

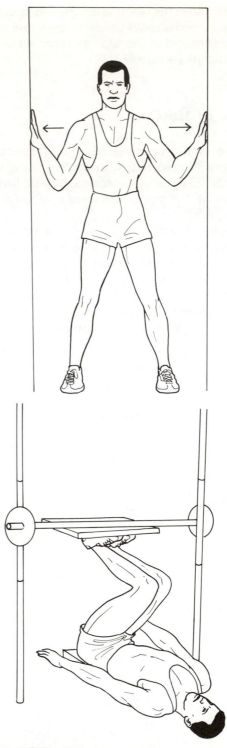

Figure 16.2.   Isometric exercises.

Isotonic Exercises

Once range of motion and some strength have been restored, strength can be more effectively developed by using isotonic exercises. When you perform an isotonic exercise, the muscle changes length and movement takes place at the joint. The necessary overload to stimulate muscle development initially may be provided by having another person offer manual resistance against the normal patterns of movement; however, such resistance should *never* be so great that movement of the part is prevented, becomes jerky, or causes pain but should be adjusted on the basis of the rehabilitating athlete's capability.

When you supervise isotonic exercises (such as the biceps curl and others illustrated in Figure 16.3), remember that the trick to gaining strength is to select a workload that is an *overload*. This overload must always remain within the muscle's capability and must be some sort of weight that can be *progressively increased*. In this way, the muscle is subjected to a workload greater than that to which it is accustomed but less than a load that could cause injury.

The body adapts to the stresses placed on it, and the muscles, tendons, ligaments, and other soft tissues thus become stronger. As the body adapts, the workload should be progressively increased so that it continues to be an overload. The key is to stress the tissues so they will adapt and not to strain them to the point of structural damage. This is a "train not strain" approach.

The DeLorme method of Progressive Resistance Exercise (see DeLorme & Watkins, 1955) is widely used during rehabilitation. It provides a safe way of overloading a muscle. A repetition (rep) is the number of times that the exercise is completed in succession. Reps are arranged in sets, which are groups of reps of

an exercise to be done with or without a rest between groups. In the DeLorme system, 3 sets of 10 reps are completed for each exercise in the rehabilitation program.

An assigned rehabilitation program will indicate a suitable weight (overload) for each exercise. This figure is called the *maximum overload* and is calculated by determining the maximum amount of weight that can be lifted only 10 times. If the weight can be lifted more than 10 times, it is too light. If it cannot be lifted 10 times, it is too heavy. The maximum overload for each exercise is initially found through a process of trial and error. In some cases, you may be asked to assist in finding this maximum overload. Progress carefully to avoid aggravating the injury.

Remember that you are dealing with an injured limb and be sure to select a relatively light workload. In fact, at first the overload may simply be the weight that produces slight fatigue on completing the 10th repetition while still being able to do the exercise correctly. In some cases, this may mean that the exercise is initially done without any weight added.

The DeLorme method progression is arranged as follows:

- 1 × 10 at ½ maximum overload
- 1 × 10 at ¾ maximum overload
- 1 × 10 at maximum overload

The first set is at ½ the athlete's maximum overload and serves as a warm-up. For example, if the maximum overload for an exercise is 20 pounds, then the athlete should first lift 10 pounds 10 times in succession. As the

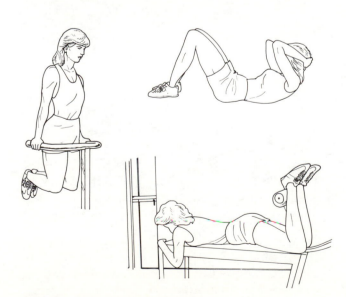
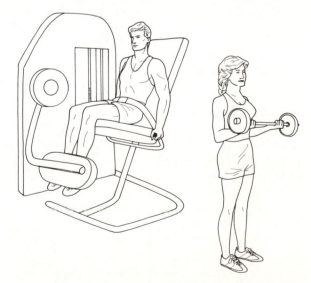

Figure 16.3.   Isotonic exercises.

athlete begins the lifts, you should emphasize the importance of doing the exercise exactly as directed and using the correct muscles. Some athletes will attempt to introduce into the lift either momentum (by lifting the weight too fast) or other, stronger muscles. This practice must be pointed out and discouraged.

In the above example, the second set of an exercise would be done at ¾ the maximum overload, or at 15 pounds. The final set would be at the maximum overload, or at 20 pounds. The athlete should stop when fatigue sets in even if all the reps cannot be completed. The goal in the third and final set (1 × 10 maximum overload) is 10 properly executed reps.

Once the third set can be done, the physician will probably recommend that the overload be increased by 1 or 2 pounds, depending on the exercise. The progression begins again; however, the athlete may not be able to execute as many reps of the exercise when this additional weight is added. Remember, the purpose of the exercise is to stress, not to strain. Adding too heavy a weight may overstress the healing tissue and result in tendinitis or another overstress injury.

As a cool-down, you may be asked to add a fourth set of 20 reps at ¼ the maximum overload (5 pounds in the example). Cooling down is just as important in rehabilitation as it is in any physical activity. In fact, it may be even more important!

The athlete should do the exercises slowly to ensure that the correct technique is used. The weight should be lifted to a count of 3, held for a count 1, and then slowly lowered back to the starting position at the count of 3. Slowly executing the exercise provides adequate time for the entire range of motion to be utilized. Slowly lowering the weights causes the same muscles that lifted the weight to continue working to control it, thus lengthening the muscles as they work and helping to build strength.

Isokinetic Exercises

The third type of strength training is the isokinetic method. It relies entirely on the use of exercise machines, although not all exercise machines are isokinetic. Isokinetics are similar to isotonics because the muscle shortens as it contracts and the joint moves. However, in isotonic exercise the resistance remains the same as the joint is moved through the range of motion. In fact, the heaviest weight that the athlete can lift is actually the amount of weight that can be lifted by the muscle in the weakest part of its range. Isokinetic machines (see Figure 16.4) continually alter the resistance so that the weight remains maximal throughout the entire range of motion prescribed by the exercise.

Isokinetic machines are widely used in general strength-training programs. Their greatest limitations are their high cost and the fact that they rarely offer the adaptability offered by free weights.

Free Weights

Whenever weights are used, special concerns must be addressed. This is true whether the

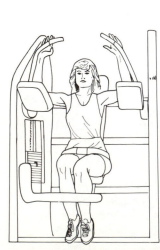 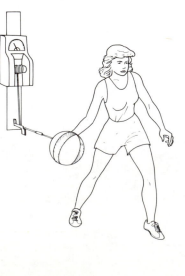 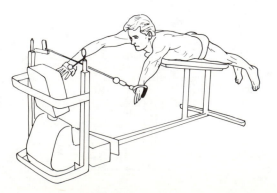

Figure 16.4. Isokinetic exercise machines.

weights are used for rehabilitation or for conditioning. Because the rehabilitating athlete is limited in what he or she can do by lack of strength and possible pain and because he or she is often not able to control the free weight as effectively as the uninjured athlete, special emphasis must be paid to every aspect of safety and the correct utilization of equipment.

The basic rules for weight training apply to rehabilitation using free weights:

- Do not use the weight room without supervision. Remember that young athletes are often tempted to experiment when left alone.
- Use spotters whenever a weight is to be lifted over the head or above the chest with the lifter in a reclining position.
- Check collars of free weights before use.
- Always wear shoes in the weight room.
- Wipe the hands dry or use chalk before grasping the bar.

The general principles of rehabilitation apply to all age groups. However, it is important that you appreciate the distinction between the strength-developing exercises that are prescribed during rehabilitation and weight training as part of a conditioning program. During rehabilitation, the primary goal is to give the injured limb the same amount of strength that it had before the injury. In a general weight training program, athletes are attempting to increase strength beyond their normal level.

This distinction must be understood by all coaches who work with preadolescent athletes. These athletes can gain strength by participating in a well-supervised strength-training program that is a part of their rehabilitation. However, these athletes are likely to be inexperienced in handling weights and will need instruction. The safest approach for rehabilitation is to use fixed-weight machines rather than free weights and to allow the athlete to complete only the exercises that have been assigned by the physician.

Muscular Endurance

Once the rehabilitating athlete gets to within 60%-80% of normal strength development, the emphasis will probably be switched to muscular endurance (i.e., the ability to continue work over a period of time). Muscular endurance is directly related to strength since strong muscles are necessary if work is to be prolonged.

To develop muscular endurance you increase the number of reps of an exercise while decreasing the overload. Endurance is developed by lifting a lighter weight many times, while strength is developed by lifting a heavy weight fewer times. The exercises are exactly the same, but the number of reps and the workload differ.

For endurance, the DeLorme method of progressive resistance exercise is modified as follows:

- 1 × 20-25 at ½ maximum overload
- 1 × 20-25 at ¾ maximum overload
- 1 × 20-25 at maximum overload
- 1 × 20-25 at ¼ maximum overload

Note that the maximum overload for muscular endurance exercises is 50% of the maximum overload used during strength rehabilitation. In our previous examples (p. 176), the maximum overload for muscular endurance exercises would be 10 pounds.

In most cases, you will be directed to follow the same guidelines for progression as were given for the strength-gaining exercises. The athlete should continue with the strength exercises, but they should be done on alternate days until normal strength is regained or as otherwise directed by the physician.

Cardiorespiratory Endurance

Cardiorespiratory endurance activities include swimming, bicycling, jogging, and running. You will probably be asked to introduce these activities at the very beginning of rehabilitation or soon after the beginning of the muscular-endurance stage of rehabilitation, depending on the nature of the injury. Have the athlete start with the least stressful of these activities based on the extremity afflicted. Individual tolerance is always the guideline. If, for example, the athlete is rehabilitating a dislocated shoulder, swimming is not recommended until his or her strength is adequate to stabilize the joint and motion is pain free. However, this same athlete can start *stationary bicycling* immediately as long as there is no discomfort and range of motion is near normal.

Riding a bicycle (freewheeling) is too dangerous. Remember, the athlete is not at his or her best, the risk of accidents greatly increases with freewheeling, and you cannot assume that the athlete has the riding skills required to keep the activity safe. You must assign stationary bicycling.

Before moving on to a walking or jogging program, the athlete must be able to hop on an injured leg (i.e, a one-foot takeoff and a one-foot landing) with no discomfort. Before the athlete is ready to try the hop, the physician will want to observe (or have you observe and report) if the athlete can

- rise up on the toes of the involved leg and hold this position for a time equal to what can be done with the uninjured leg, or
- jump with a one- or two-foot takeoff and land on both feet.

You should start the athlete with a slow jog on an even surface and alternate this with a walk. Build up the distance without changing speed, then slowly increase speed. Progression should follow this format:

1. Run straight ahead at ½ speed
2. Run straight ahead at ¾ speed
3. Run straight ahead at full speed
4. Run and cut

WARNING:

Do *not* use ankle weights during walking, jogging, or running to increase the overload on the muscles as they can cause a whiplash effect and may impose too much stress on the recovering tissues.

Rehabilitation of a knee injury should include swimming, bicycling, and jogging, progressing in that order. Swimming should be introduced when the athlete can successfully execute 3 sets of 20 straight-leg raises with an overload of 10%-15% of the body weight. Overloads of 15% should be used only with athletes who have completed the growth spurt, which indicates that the growth plates have closed.

By the time swimming is introduced, the athlete should be beginning flexion/extension exercises. At first, have the athlete kick with straight legs using the flutter kick. Later, as the range of motion and strength improve, the thigh muscles will receive more exercise if the flutter kick is continued but is done with a bent-knee action.

When the athlete begins stationary bicycling, the speed of pedaling should be increased as discomfort decreases. Set the tension at a level where the athlete can maintain a "speed" of 90-120 revolutions per minutes for 5 minutes. Slowly increase the exercise time to 10 minutes. By bicycling rapidly (or by kicking rapidly when swimming), the athlete is "teaching" the muscles to contract quickly. This type of muscle activity is essential in most sports.

During the early stages of knee rehabilitation, the kneecap is very vulnerable and prone to irritation. Make certain that you have properly adjusted the bicycle seat to allow for near complete extension of the knee. The knee should not lock in the fully extended position.

Do not let the athlete jog until he or she can lift 80% of the body weight once using the injured leg only. The athlete must be able to go from at least 90° flexion at the knee to a full extension. Some coaches ask athletes to perform a series of one leg squats on the injured leg. This procedure is effective, but may lead to reinjury as athletes go too far in their flexion.

If you have the use of a pool, you can easily determine whether an athlete with a lower extremity injury is ready to jog by having the athlete jog in chest deep water. If the individual experiences no pain, he or she may begin jogging.

Agility and Coordination (Skill)

You will be instructed to add agility exercises to the program once the athlete can run straight ahead at full speed without discomfort. The best way to improve agility is to have the athlete perform activities that require quick starts, stops, and changes in direction.

Begin with gradual changes of direction, such as running circles and figure eights, then progress through the following activities: starts and stops; backward, sideways, and crossover runs; zigzag runs; and right-angle cuts. Finally, you should add coordination and skill exercises that are directly related to the athlete's particular sport. For example, in baseball you would use throwing, catching, batting, and running the bases to help regain the athlete's preinjury ability level.

An important phase of lower extremity rehabilitation is often overlooked—retraining the receptors in the body (proprioceptors) that transmit information concerning the body position in space. Proper functioning of the receptors is necessary to prevent recurring injuries.

The progression for retraining these receptors is as follows:

- Sitting with the involved foot on a balance board (a 2-foot circle made from ¾-inch plywood mounted on ⅔ of a croquet ball), balance the board. This apparatus or a similar device must be approved by the attending physician.
- Seated, touch with the involved foot five or six small pieces of tape randomly arranged in a 1-foot square.
- Stand on the involved foot with eyes open.
- Stand on the involved foot with eyes closed.
- Bounce on a minitramp. (Not all athletes will receive physician's approval for this activity.)
- Hop from side to side, forward and back, and diagonally.
- Balance on the balance board with both feet. Progress to balancing on one foot.

The final decision to allow the athlete to return to full activity rests with the attending physician. You should let the physician know whether all the rehabilitation activities have been performed successfully. Once the athlete returns to full activity, you should

- apply heat before activity to stimulate circulation at the injury site, and
- apply ice after activity to control any swelling.

GENERAL PROGRAM GUIDELINES

To be effective, the rehabilitation program must be followed daily until the athlete meets all the requirements for returning to activity that were set up by the attending physician. At that time you may be directed to reduce the schedule to 3 days per week.

In most cases, the best person to detect problems with the rehabilitation program is the athlete. Make certain that the athlete understands the significance of pain and swelling. Instruct him or her to look for swelling in the morning and again in the evening. Swelling that occurs during the day and is gone the next morning is normal when tissue is recovering. However, swelling that is present in the morning indicates too much activity.

As soon as you are informed of any increase in pain and/or swelling, contact the attending physician. You may be directed to cut back on the athlete's activity level, or if necessary, curtail the athlete's daily program until the physician can reevaluate the entire rehabilitation schedule. Remember, progression is set by the healing of the body tissues and the individual's tolerance to the workload.

WARNING:

Any significant increase in swelling or pain or the additional loss of range of motion, strength, or endurance means that the athlete must be reexamined by a physician.

SUMMARY AND RECOMMENDATIONS

Stress on an injured body part must be minimal during healing. Total inactivity is not the answer. Instead, there must be a link between healing and full recovery—a rehabilitation program.

1. The primary goals of rehabilitation are to restore the injured part to the level of function required by the athlete's particular activity and to ensure that strength, flexibility, and endurance are returned to preinjury levels.
2. Five key physical factors can be diminished as a result of injury. These are range of motion, strength, muscular endurance, cardiorespiratory endurance, and skill (agility and coordination).
3. A rehabilitation program is a systematic approach to restoring the five factors and begins with range of motion and ends with skill.

4. The program cannot begin without the approval of the attending physician.
5. The guideline for proceeding from one stage of rehabilitation to the next is *normality*.
6. Rehabilitation should not cause additional pain or swelling. The rehabilitation program's schedule is set by the healing of body tissue and the individual's tolerance to the workload.
7. The final decision of returning the athlete to full participation rests with the attending physician.

Chapter 17
Heat and Cold Therapy

Any therapeutic aid used in the treatment of an injury is called a *modality*. Selecting the proper modality and applying it correctly will help provide the best practical environment for healing. However, if the injured and surrounding tissues are overstimulated by a modality that is applied too frequently or too intensely, the result can be harmful. Tissues may swell and pain may increase, often prolonging the healing process.

The improper application of a treatment modality is often related to a desire to accelerate healing. If you start the modality too soon, apply it for too long a period of time, or repeat the treatment too often, your actions will usually lead to delayed or improper healing. The old axiom that time heals all wounds has its place in the treatment of athletic injuries. The modalities that you will use do *not* accelerate healing but promote it. If you attempt to accelerate the healing process, it can only be delayed.

The choice of using heat or cold is usually not a difficult one. However, if an athlete has any loss of sensation in the body part to be treated, neither modality should be used. You should not use heat if swelling is still taking place or if there are indications of inflammation. Skin color and temperature can be used as a simple check for when to use heat. If the skin is redder or deeper in color than the surrounding tissues, stay with cold treatments until the color at the injury site is the same as that of the surrounding skin. If the injured part feels warmer than the surrounding skin or the corresponding uninjured part, there may still be bleeding taking place at the injury site. In such cases, continue with cold therapy. New muscle and joint inflammations are best cared for with cold therapies.

When you are in doubt about the application of a modality, consult the attending physician. Usually, treatment begins with cold therapy; heat therapy will be delayed for 72 hours after the injury.

WARNING:

Do *not* apply cold or heat therapies to open injuries.

COLD THERAPIES

The application of cold therapy, also called *cryotherapy*, is the primary means of reducing the swelling and inflammation associated with most athletic injuries. The RICE method described on page 63 is the initial treatment for the majority of closed injuries that are free of possible fractures or severe joint injury. Cold therapy may take the form of ice packs, gel packs, ice massage, ice slush, or cold-water immersion.

Applying Cold

When cold is applied, the initial reaction is a lowered temperature at the injury site and in the surrounding tissues, which will decrease tissue damage. The body's first response to this cooling is to reduce nerve impulses from the injury site. Thus the cold acts as an *anesthetic*. During this same time period, nerve impulses in the affected muscles are reduced, leading to a reduction of muscle spasms. Blood flow into the cooled area is decreased as capillaries constrict and will result in a reduction of bleeding at the injury site. The application of cold also will lower cell activities (metabolism). With a decreased metabolic rate, a cell requires less oxygen to carry out its functions and to survive. Following an injury, the availability of oxygen may be disrupted, causing additional tissue destruction and the accompanying swelling. Cooling the area (with ice) will decrease the cell's need for oxygen when it may not be readily available, thus reducing swelling.

During the first 5 minutes, athletes will experience a range of sensations. The following sensations are normal and should not terminate a treatment:

- Coldness
- Burning
- Tingling
- Stinging or aching
- Numbness

Specific Cold Modalities

Cold therapy should be applied to the closed injury area for the first 48-72 hours after injury. The application time will vary depending on the form of cold therapy that is being used. Cold therapy can be applied by the athlete at home with little preparation or mess. The major difficulty is the discomfort first experienced when the cold is applied. The same precautions used with the RICE method also apply to other forms of cold therapy (see p. 63).

Ice Packs

Ice packs can be used alone or with compression and elevation when appropriate. An ice pack can be made quickly by placing ice chips or cubes into a moist towel. This method should not be used if the athlete is exposed to a harsh environment while the cold is being applied. A better system is to use a heavy-duty plastic bag to hold the ice as this will prevent moisture from contacting the injury site and prevent the mess that will occur as the ice melts. A "ziplock" type of plastic bag is useful since it allows for the easy draining of water as the ice melts. Regardless of the type of plastic bag that is used, a moist cloth cover should be

wrapped around the bag (see Figure 17.1) to improve comfort and to help reduce excessive cold reaching the athlete's skin. In extremely cold environments, wrap the plastic with a dry cloth or towel to reduce the possibility of frostbite. If ice is to be applied to the eye, wrap the ice bag with a dry cloth.

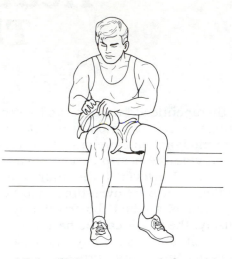

Figure 17.1. Using an ice pack for cold therapy.

The ice pack should be applied for 20-30 minutes. Compression and elevation should be maintained after the pack is removed. The ice pack can be reapplied every 90 minutes throughout the day and evening. Be aware, however, that a good night's sleep is more important to recovery than applying ice during the night.

Gel and Chemical Cold Packs

Commercial flexible silicone gel cold packs are available at most drug stores and require less preparation than other forms of cold therapy and prove to be less messy for the athlete to use. Before using the gel pack, it should be placed in a freezer for 15-20 minutes. A new pack may take 1-2 hours to cool sufficiently. Do not attempt to cool a heat pack and use this for cold therapy as it will become too stiff when frozen to allow it to conform to the shape of the body part.

The flexible gel cold pack is convenient to use; however, the packs get colder than ice (below 0 °F), which means that frostbite could occur if care is not exercised. To protect the tissues, wrap the cooled pack in a damp towel before applying it to the skin, and keep it in place for no more than 20-30 minutes. Use a dry towel to cover the pack in a cold environment. The gel pack can be used alone or with compression and elevation.

As the pack warms, do not exchange it for a newly frozen one. Instead, keep it in place for the full time of treatment. Return the pack to the freezer to cool for reuse. Should the pack's plastic cover tear, you can mend it with vinyl tape. The tape should be applied to a clean, dry surface to ensure a good seal. If necessary, a new cover can be purchased at a drug store or medical supply house, or the pack can be placed in a large, heavy-duty Ziploc plastic bag.

Commercial chemical cold packs are manufactured to allow for the quick mixing of chemicals to produce cold. Although they appear to be a quick and easy way to apply cold therapy, you should be aware of the problems associated with their use. Many athletic trainers have complained that these cold packs vary significantly in the amount of cold produced and do not always remain cold long enough to allow for the completion of the therapy. Also, if a chemical cold pack leaks or bursts (rare), its chemicals could produce skin burns. In addition to these problems, the coach who wishes to use chemical cold packs should realize that they are expensive and can be used only once.

Ice Massage

This technique involves massaging the injury site and surrounding areas with ice. It is most useful in the early stages of rehabilitation, when the athlete is attempting to regain normal range of motion. The advantage of ice massage over cold packs is that the cold will penetrate more deeply into the tissues. Consequently, pain relief and muscle relaxation are enhanced.

Ice massage is not meant to be used immediately following an injury. Because freshly injured tissues may benefit from compression and elevation, and because more tissue comes in contact with an ice pack for a longer period of time, the RICE method is a better choice of action immediately following an injury. Once the athlete is responding well to repeated ice-pack therapy, the ice massage may be a useful part of rehabilitation. Its use should, however, be approved by the attending physician.

To prepare the ice for an ice massage, freeze water in styrofoam or paper cups (see Figure

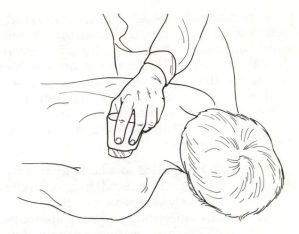

Figure 17.2. Water can be frozen in a styrofoam cup to provide the source of cold for an ice massage.

17.2). Styrofoam may be preferable because it will insulate the massager's fingers from the cold. Cut or tear away a bit of the cup's edge to expose about 1 inch of ice, and continue to do this as the ice melts. Massage the injury site by gently rubbing the ice on the athlete's skin, using small circles or back-and-forth strokes and making certain to wipe any water from the athlete's skin to facilitate cooling. At first, the athlete's muscles may tighten as a temporary reaction to the sudden, intense cooling. Do not stop the treatment. During the first 5 minutes of massaging, the athlete should experience a full range of sensations as noted on page 184. Massage the injury site until numbness occurs, usually 8-10 minutes. Stop the treatment when numbness occurs or when the skin color brightens (e.g., white to bright pink).

Once the injured area is numb, the athlete should begin range-of-motion exercises but only through the pain free range. Do not apply force. Continue this exercise for about 3 minutes. If possible, the ice massage should be repeated with the exercise cycle two more times. This treatment of three cycles of ice massage and exercise may be repeated two or three times a day. Discontinue the treatment once the normal range of motion has been regained.

Ice Slush

Immersion of the injured part in a mixture of cold water and ice can be used for cold therapy if approved by the attending physician. Usually, the physician will allow an ice-slush treatment to begin immediately following a closed injury to the hand, foot, or ankle if there are no indications of open wounds, moderate to severe internal bleeding, severe swelling, or severe sprains or strains. While the injured part is immersed, the athlete can execute range-of-motion exercises, utilizing the buoyant effect of the water and its resistance to motion.

Ice slush offers three advantages over other forms of cold therapy:

- Cold can be applied to a large area of the body (e.g., an entire hand, foot, or ankle).
- The entire body part is cooled uniformly as the slush conforms to the body anatomy.
- The cold penetrates more deeply than with other cold therapies.

The major disadvantage of ice-slush immersion is that it is the most painful method of applying cold. Other disadvantages include the need for a large container, increased discomfort if used with compression, and not being able to use elevation.

For a new injury, the ice-slush bath should be between 45°F and 65°F. The ice-slush treatment is set up by filling a large container with water and enough ice cubes or chips to lower the temperature to the desired level. The injured part should be immersed entirely on the first attempt even though there will be some discomfort. The athlete should keep the injured part submerged until it is numb or until he or she is unable to tolerate the cold. If necessary, the athlete can take the part out of the slush momentarily to warm it. The in-and-out pattern should be continued, as necessary, until numbness sets in but should last no longer than 20 minutes. As an added safety precaution, someone should stay with the athlete during the treatment to reduce chances of overexposure to cold and to guard against the rare possibility of the athlete fainting in response to the shock of the intense cold.

> **WARNING:**
>
> If the ice-slush treatment is taking place in a whirlpool bath, do *not* turn on the turbine. The circulating water will drastically reduce the temperature, making frostbite a distinct possibility. Also, the action of the water may cause additional injury to healing tissues. Do *not* add salt to the slush mixture.

HEAT THERAPIES

Applying heat to a closed injury site is a time-tested form of therapy. Great care must be exercised in its use since there is a danger of burning tissues when heat therapy is improperly applied. Always supervise heat treatments. Also, be aware that individuals react differently to heat. Make certain that you use individual tolerance as a guide (fair-skinned and/or light-haired people are usually more sensitive to heat than those with darker pigmentations). Explain to the athlete that therapeutic heat should be comfortably warm and soothing and not hot.

As you instruct the athlete, be certain that you discourage the idea that if a little is good, more must be better. This belief only encourages a toleration of discomfort, with the result being the development of first- and second-degree burns. You should keep checking the athlete during the heat treatment to determine if the treated area is becoming too warm. Ask the athlete if the treated area feels hot and look for skin-color changes (e.g., red coloration) that indicate a buildup of heat. If the area becomes too warm, stop the treatment or adjust the temperature to which the athlete is being exposed. This may require utilizing a different heat modality or discontinuing heat therapy entirely for the day.

Applying Heat

The application of heat will promote muscle relaxation and pain relief. This soothing quality of heat therapy continues only as long as the heat modality warms the tissues. While this is occurring, there is an increased flow of blood at the injury site. Blood vessels in and below the skin will increase in diameter to allow a greater flow of blood into and out of the injured area that will carry more nutrients and oxygen to the damaged tissues and carry away the waste products produced by the tissues. Because the metabolic rate is increased by heat therapy—creating a greater demand for nutrients, oxygen, and waste-product removal—this is a very important factor. The increased rate of metabolism produced during heat therapy will help enhance healing.

Heat therapy can be very beneficial to healing for certain types of injury; however, there are seven situations in which heat should *never* be used:

- When the injury site has an open wound (Heat therapy applied to open wounds may cause contamination and injury to the tissues at the site.)
- When bleeding and swelling have not been controlled (The increased blood flow will cause additional blood loss from damaged capillaries and other blood vessels and may restart serious bleeding. Even if the bleeding itself is not serious, the seepage of blood will cause an increase of swelling at the injury site.)
- When sensation is impaired (The athlete cannot tell if the tissue is burning if the heat cannot be felt.)
- When circulation is congested, as in a moderate to severe bruise (The congestion prevents the body from regulating tissue temperature, mainly by hindering the flow of normal temperature blood into the treated area to replace that which has been warmed. The result is that the tissues could be burned.)
- When tissues are extremely sensitive to heat (This is particularly true of the eyes and of the entire genital region.)
- When the injury is recent (Do *not* use heat treatment until approximately 48-72 hours after the injury has occurred. This will give time for swelling and internal bleeding to be controlled and initial wound healing to be strong enough to prevent the reopening of wounds.)
- When metal is embedded in the skin or underlying structures (If the athlete has surgical pins or clips, screws, or metal plates under or adjacent to the injury site, do *not* apply heat therapy. The metal may absorb heat, increasing the danger of deep-tissue burning.) This warning applies primarily to "deep heat" modalities, such as ultrasound, which penetrate deeply underneath skin. In addition, metal on the surface of the skin (jewelry) that is heated may cause superficial burns.

WARNING:

Always remove all metal objects on the surface of the skin prior to applying heat therapy. This includes watches, necklaces, earrings, bracelets, hooks, and snaps.

Table 17.1
The Effects of Cold and Heat Therapy

Indicant	Cold therapy	Heat therapy
Pain	↓	↓
Muscle spasms	↓	↓
Blood flow	↓	↑

Table 17.1 compares the effects of cold and heat therapy. An arrow pointing up (↑) signifies an increase, while one pointing down (↓) signifies a decrease.

Specific Heat Modalities

There are several superficial (penetrating not much deeper than a point just below the skin surface) heat modalities that can be used at home as well as in the training room. These treatments include heated-water soaks, heat packs, heating pads, and analgesic packs. Again, make certain that the athlete understands how to limit his or her exposure to excessive heat before you recommend any home heat therapy. In addition, the athlete should be told to limit exposure to the heat treatment to no more than 15-20 minutes.

Heated Water Soaks

Although most individuals can tolerate water that is up to 113°F for 10-20 minutes, it is best to immerse the injured part in water that is no hotter than 102°F to 104°F. This will keep the water in a comfortable, safe range and will provide the desired benefits of therapy. During the treatment, the athlete should move the injured part slowly through its pain free range of motion.

Heat Packs

A heat pack is usually a canvas bag that has been filled with silicated gel. Packs of various sizes can be purchased at most drugstores. Care must be taken when applying the pack to avoid exposing the athlete's skin to excessive heat. In addition to this problem, the weight of the pack on top of an injury site may prove to be too uncomfortable for the injured athlete. Avoid placing a heat pack on top of a sensitive or tender injury site. Always check with the athlete to be certain that there is no discomfort once the pack is in place.

It is easy to prepare a heat pack for use. Simply immerse it completely in a pan of water and bring the water to a boil. Once this occurs, turn the heat to low and allow 20-30 minutes for the pack to absorb the heat. It is a good idea to check the water temperature periodically during this time to make certain that it stays at or slightly below 160°F. If the pack has never been used before, let it soak in water overnight before heating the water or hold the 160°F soak for several hours.

Once the pack has been heated, allow the excess surface water to drip off and then wrap the pack in several layers of toweling (see Figure 17.3). Two towels will usually be enough; however, some athletes may request an additional wrap for comfort (a special terry-cloth cover is available for covering the pack). Fold each towel in half lengthwise and place one on top of the other so that they crisscross. Put the pack in the center and fold the ends so that six to eight layers of towels are on the top of the pack.

The thickest side of the covered pack should be placed next to the athlete's skin. Remind the athlete that discomfort due to excessive heat indicates that the pack is too hot. Be certain that you warn the athlete not to build up excessive heat by lying on the pack. Once the pack is in place, lay an additional towel over the top of it to help prevent heat loss.

The heat pack should be kept in place for 15-20 minutes. Do *not* exchange the pack for a newly heated one as it cools as this will greatly increase the chances of the treatment's leading to skin burns. Instead, remove or add layers of toweling to adjust the heat reaching the athlete's skin. If the treatment is to be repeated frequently, return the pack to the pan of hot water for short-term storage. Whenever the pack must be reheated for use, remember to turn the heat to low once the water begins to boil.

When storing a heat pack, place it in an airtight plastic bag and put it in a freezer (not in a refrigerator) to help prevent the growth of bacteria and mold. Thaw the pack before it is to be reheated. If the pack dries out (the silicate gel hardens), you can restore it by soaking the pack in water until the gel softens. Once this has been done, the pack may be reheated. Note that drying will eventually shorten the life of the pack.

Electrical Moist Heating Pads

Another superficial heat modality that is convenient to use at home (and perhaps is less of a bother than the standard heat pack) is an electrical moist heating pad. This type of device, available at most drugstores, is a thermostatically controlled pad with a sealed plastic covering that is approved for moist usage. Make certain that the athlete follows the manufacturer's directions and that the device is UL approved and has a "dead man's" switch to insure that the heating pad turns off if the athlete falls asleep. Typically, the pad should be applied to the injured area for 15-20 minutes while being set on medium.

WARNING:

Inform the athlete that this is a *special* type of heating pad. Caution him or her not to attempt to use a standard pad and moist towels!

Analgesic Pack

Analgesic rubs and packs are used by many coaches and trainers, with some of these individuals going so far as to create their own "secret mixtures." Studies have shown that these compounds are very limited in their ability to penetrate and may actually act as irritants, which cause blistering of the skin. For

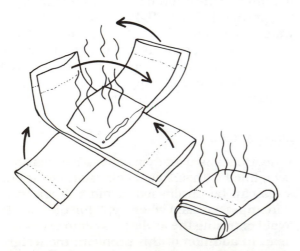

Figure 17.3. Two towels can be used to wrap a heat pack prior to its application.

the coach who disagrees with these conclusions and wishes to use analgesics, this section is presented to serve as a guideline for safe application.

Preparations containing oil of wintergreen (methyl salicylate) can be rubbed on the skin as therapy for sore muscles and stiff joints prior to activity. The result is a warm and soothing effect that is produced from the dilation of superficial blood vessels. Such preparations should never be used on new joint or muscle injuries.

Analgesic balms come in different strengths and with different bases, but the most common is methyl salicylate. Oil-based products are likely to stain clothing and may prove to be difficult to remove from the skin. If an oil-based product is used and proves to be too hot for the athlete, hot water must be used to remove the balm, thus making the area even hotter. The best course of action is to use a water-soluble balm. If the athlete complains of too much heat being generated during treatment, cool water will remove this type of balm and will help reduce the excessive heat.

Once the balm is placed on the skin over the top of a closed-injury site, you can cover the area with an insulator to intensify and prolong the effect of the heat being generated. This technique is called an *analgesic pack*. It allows for the athlete to benefit from the effects of the balm during activity.

Do *not* precede the use of analgesic balms with other forms of heat therapy. If a physician has recommended that heat therapy and balms be used, wait at least 15 minutes after the heat therapy before applying a balm or balm pack to avoid blistering the athlete's skin.

If an athlete who is wearing an analgesic pack complains that it is getting too hot, remove the pack immediately and wash the area with mildly soapy water. If blistering occurs, stop using the balm and have the athlete seen by a physician.

WARNING:

Never apply an analgesic balm around the eyes, mucous membranes, or open wounds.

When preparing an analgesic pack, rub a thin layer of *mild* analgesic balm into the skin over the injury site. If there is tenderness at the site that makes this procedure painful, stop at once. Only *small areas* of skin should receive the application of balm.

Be aware that weather conditions may influence the effectiveness of the balm. An increase in temperature or humidity will increase the absorption of the balm and intensify the heating effect. Under hot or very humid conditions, the athlete may not be able to tolerate the analgesic pack and is best treated using the balm without any insulating coverings.

Once the balm has been properly applied to the athlete's skin, cover the area with a clean layer of toweling, cotton sheeting, or a disposable baby diaper. Secure the covering in place with an elastic bandage, which should run from the bottom edge of the covering to the top edge in a herringbone pattern. Secure the edge by taping. Do not use pins or clips since they may open during activity and injure the athlete or another player.

A disposable baby diaper makes the best covering for the analgesic pack because it has a plastic shield that prevents the balm from penetrating through to the bandage. In addition, the balm penetrates more deeply and the athlete experiences a greater heating effect due to the occlusive nature of the diaper. The same effect can be achieved by placing a plastic wrap over the outside of the toweling before applying the elastic bandage wrap.

During activity analgesic packs tend to slip. To alleviate this problem spray the adjacent, uninjured areas with tape adherent before applying the elastic bandage. The adherent will help secure the bandage. In addition, if the pack is being applied to the thigh, loop the bandage around the waist once to create a figure-eight pattern.

CONTRAST BATHS

A contrast bath may be used to provide a treatment that causes alternating periods of blood-vessel dilation and constriction at and near the injury site. A contrast bath should be used only at the stage when both bleeding and swelling have been controlled. Its main use is for cases in which swelling is controlled but remains constant despite therapeutic attempts at reduction. In all these cases, the athlete should first be examined by a physician, and the contrast bath should be the recommendation of the physician.

To set up a contrast bath, you will need two large plastic containers, several towels, two thermometers, a timer or clock, and a stool or chair. Fill one of the containers three-fourths full with 104 °F water. Put cold water in the second container and cool this bath by adding ice cubes until the temperature is between 55 °F and 65 °F. Allow adequate room for the immersion of the injured limb so that overflow will not occur.

First, immerse the injured part in the cold water for 1 minute, then switch immediately to the warm water for 5 minutes. Repeat this process a total of five times and end with the cold-water treatment. The blood vessels will constrict with the final immersion, thus reducing the possibility of additional swelling. This treatment can be done several times a day.

If the contrast bath is to be followed by a massage, end the treatment with a hot-water immersion. This will leave the blood vessels dilated and thus improve the effects of the massage.

SUMMARY AND RECOMMENDATIONS

The primary treatment modalities that can be applied by coaches and athletes are heat and cold therapies. Do *not* apply heat or cold therapies to open injuries or when bleeding has not been controlled. Make certain that you always guard against frostbite or tissue burning.

1. In most cases, cold can be used to reduce swelling and inflammation.
2. Cold therapy may take the form of ice packs, gels packs, ice massage, or ice-slush immersion baths.
3. Cold therapies should be limited to no more than 20-30 minutes of application. Applications may be repeated after 90 minutes.
4. Heat therapy should be adjusted to the athlete's heat tolerance and must *always* be monitored to help prevent tissue burning.
5. Common treatments include heated-water soaks, heat packs, heating pads, and analgesic packs.
6. Cold therapy may be applied to most closed injuries for the first 48-72 hours after injury. Heat treatments may be applied after that time. However, you should *not* use heat therapy if swelling is still taking place or if there are other signs of inflammation.

Chapter 18
Exercise Equipment in Rehabilitation

The use of weights as part of a physician-approved rehabilitation program often gives the coach a chance to participate directly with the injured athlete. Even when the physician utilizes a physical therapist or athletic trainer, certain exercises involving weights are assigned to be done away from medical offices and facilities, giving the coach a chance to supervise the activity. It is the coach's responsibility to keep the athlete from attempting too much too soon.

WEIGHT-TRAINING EQUIPMENT

There are two major types of weight training equipment (see Figure 18.1):

- Weight-training machines (weights that are secured and guided by cables)
- Free weights (metal discs, collars, and bars of different sizes that can be made into barbells or dumbbells of different total weights)

Weight-training machines are usually safer and easier to use than free weights and are necessary for the isokinetic exercises that are suggested in rehabilitation and conditioning programs. Many of the machines commonly available to the coach are isotonic machines and are less suited for rehabilitation exercises (e.g., Universal Gyms). If you intend to use isotonic machines for rehabilitation, you must exercise great care in assigning overloads and developing range of motion. Due to the high cost of isotonic and isokinetic machines, the use of free weights may be the only affordable method of regaining muscular strength and endurance.

Free weights offer a greater range of exercise versatility in comparison to that which is available with a machine. The major difficulty with free weights is that they are entirely controlled by the athlete using them. It is very easy for an injured athlete who is trying to regain muscle strength by using free weights to aggravate the original injury. Likewise, it is possible for this same injured athlete to reinjure healed tissues

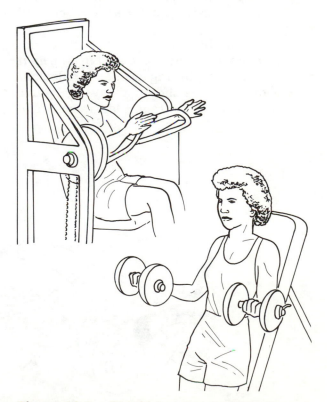

Figure 18.1. Weight-training equipment.

by overestimating the amount of weight that can be controlled or lifted without harm. In addition to these problems, the athlete may sustain new injuries through improper lifting techniques. You can help reduce the possibility of new or recurring injuries by instructing athletes in the safety precautions they should take when lifting weights.

An example of a free weight is the iron boot. This type of weight is frequently used in the early stages of knee rehabilitation (see Figure 18.2). The boot is controlled and guided by muscular strength, with stress being placed on the athlete's knee joint and supportive muscles. Even though this is a very effective piece of rehabilitation equipment, you should be wary of using the iron boot too early in the program.

The progression of exercises is very important. The athlete should begin with straight-leg raises before attempting flexion/extension exercises. If the athlete begins flexion/extension exercises too early in the program, the muscles may not have developed enough to control the rotation of the knee joint, and reinjury may occur. Equally important, the anterior thigh muscles may not be strong enough to guide the kneecap smoothly along the patellar surface of the femur. As a result, the athlete may begin to experience a painful grating sensation behind the kneecap when the knee is bent and straightened.

There is another caution that must be considered when using the iron boot: *Lift only light weights*. The beginning weight for flexion/ extension exercises should always be lighter than that used for straight-leg raises. The maximum weight for both boot and bar should never exceed 20 pounds for the adult athlete and is determined based on the athlete's body size and age. The maximum weight for younger athletes should be much less and should be strictly limited by what the attending physician requests. In flexion/extension exercises, the boot can be used to strengthen the quadriceps muscles (see Figure 18.3). When used for this purpose, the athlete should be seated on a table and the boot rested on a stool or the athlete should sit on a bench so that the weight can be easily returned to the floor. *Never* let the athlete's leg hang over a table without support being under the boot as joint and ligament injury will probably result from the undue stress placed on the ligaments of the knee.

If free weights are to be used in a rehabilitation program, the coach must know what weights to use, when to use them, what exercises are to be used, the order of the exercises, and how to perform the exercises. This information must come from the attending physician.

The proper use of free weights is a skill. If you plan to let your athletes use free weights as part of their rehabilitation programs, you must have a basic understanding of human movement (kinesiology), lifting techniques, the exercises, and the *overload principle*.

The overload principle involves increasing the strenuousness of an exercise by progressively increasing the weight used or the number of reps so that the exercise represents the maximal or near maximal performance for the athlete. Remember that the maximal perfor-

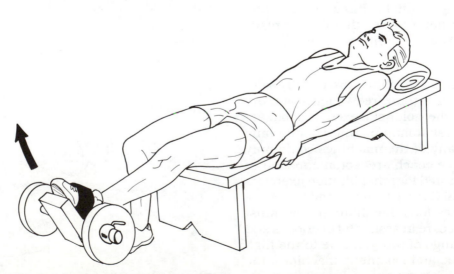

Figure 18.2. The iron boot can be used to rehabilitate an injured knee.

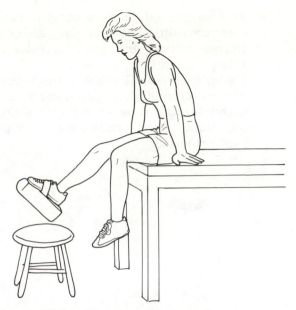

Figure 18.3. The use of the iron boot in rehabilitating the quadriceps muscles.

mance of an athlete in rehabilitation may be significantly lower than when his or her muscles are fully recovered.

You must also know how each lift is properly executed to avoid injuries. The use of free weights by your athletes requires you to explain techniques and safety measures properly to the athletes and to supervise their activities.

IMPROVISED EQUIPMENT

A coach with a limited budget needs only a little imagination to be able to improvise safe weights from inexpensive and easily acquired materials. In some cases, the program assigned by the attending physician will include suggestions on making improvised weights. The following paragraphs explain some simple ways that you can make your own weight-training equipment. The use of any equipment, however, should be approved by the physician.

Sandbags

Sandbags can be used to provide an overload in the rehabilitation of ankle, knee, wrist, elbow, and shoulder injuries. You can use any kind of heavy cloth such as canvas, cotton duck cloth, denim, or ticking to make the bags that will hold the sand. Even strong pillow-

cases can be used. The bags should be double stitched for durability.

You should also make a saddlebag to hold the sandbags. In place of the saddlebag, an old purse or a small plastic bucket will suffice. Make certain that you pad the handle of the saddlebag or other devices you use to hold the sandbags. Velcro straps can be used to hold single bags in place.

You can get sand from hardware stores, building material dealers, concrete supply houses, nurseries, pet shops, and some toy stores (very expensive!). Beach sand is also an acceptable source, but it should be washed thoroughly and dried completely before using. Make the sandbags in varying weights. A complete set should range from 1 to 10 pounds; however, you may prefer to make them in 1- or 2-pound sizes for easier control.

Seal the sand in durable plastic bags and then enclose these bags in the cloth sandbag coverings to prevent leakage through the cloth. Ziploc bags may be used as sandbags, but it is best to use two at a time, one inside the other. Unlike the cloth bags, the ziplock closings will not hold if you attempt to loop the plastic bags over the leg, so you will have to place them into a saddlebag or a similar device.

A shoebox full of clean sand is another useful piece of rehabilitation equipment. Athletes can exercise injured fingers and hands by opening and closing their hands in the sand.

Socks

A pair of tube socks stuffed with full cans and having the cuffs tied together in a square knot can make a pair of weights to be looped over the leg for ankle, shin splint, or knee exercises.

Plastic Bottles

Plastic bottles provide an inexpensive alternative to iron dumbbells for upper-extremity rehabilitation. The best kind of bottles to use are those with handles or those that narrow in the middle (e.g., detergent bottles). Such bottles are easy to grasp. You can use sand or water to provide the necessary weight. Water makes it easier to estimate the weight since 1 cup of water is equal to about ½ pound.

SUMMARY
AND RECOMMENDATIONS

Weight training is a valuable rehabilitation activity. Equipment may include weight-training machines and free weights. Consider the following in implementing rehabilitation programs:

1. The weight-training machines are safer and easier to use, but isokinetic machines are not affordable for most programs.

2. Free weights offer a great range of exercise versatility; however, they are controlled entirely by the athlete using them.

3. If your athletes will use weights as part of their rehabilitation, you must understand human movement, safe lifting techniques, the exercises, and the overload principle.

Chapter 19
Therapeutic Taping

Taping can be a useful part of a rehabilitation program; however, it should never be used to replace the program. If an athlete's muscles and ligaments are not strong enough to support a joint during activity, it is foolish to think that a layer or two of tape will provide the additional strength.

New injuries should *never* be taped. Rather, taping should be used only during the last part of rehabilitation, when the athlete is ready to return to physical activity. It is during this stage of rehabilitation that taping can provide the extra support and protection required to allow safe participation.

You must make certain that the attending physician approves of taping and the return to activity. Do not add taping on your own even if the athlete has been given his or her physician's consent to participate. Since taping is considered to be part of rehabilitation, its application must be physician-approved.

THE PURPOSES OF TAPING

Countless athletes have gone into sporting events with limbs taped, hoping to prevent injuries. Until recently, the merit of taping as a preventive measure has gone unquestioned; however, there is no evidence to show that taping is of any value in injury prevention. No one has been able to prove conclusively that tape will or will not support a muscle or a joint to the extent necessary to prevent injury. For this reason, efforts at taping should be concentrated on therapeutic taping.

The two purposes of therapeutic taping are

- to limit range of motion (the painful or injurious part of the range is avoided, pro-

tecting the recovering tissues from stress and reinjury), and
- to support healing tissues, reducing the chances of reinjury and restricting the movement of the wound edges, thus allowing healing to be uninterrupted by the effects of movement.

No two injuries to the same joint are alike; therefore, there is no one correct method of wrapping or strapping a specific joint. This is why you will find references showing dozens of patterns for taping the ankle or for dealing with chronic shin splints. Applying tape is an art. It requires a basic knowledge of human anatomy and kinesiology (the science of movement) joined with an understanding of the purposes of taping so that the person doing the taping can select the correct pattern to meet the specific needs of the injured athlete.

As a coach, you will be able to select the correct pattern for therapeutic taping if you remember the purposes of taping and consider the injury site. Remember that an injury to a muscle group will probably affect the joints above and below the site and that an injury to a joint will affect muscles above and below the joint. Always consider the anatomy of the injury site. Many different anatomical structures are probably involved in an injury. A sprain may involve stretched, torn, or ruptured ligaments or a damaged joint capsule, bone ends, blood vessels, and nerves.

BASIC MATERIALS

Various inexpensive and commonly available materials can be used in therapeutic taping. As a coach, you should know how to use all these materials and be prepared to teach the athlete the procedures required for correct application. You should do the taping; however, taping sessions provide an excellent opportunity to instruct the athlete in self-care.

Elastic Bandages

The elastic bandage used in athletics is a cotton wrap reinforced with rubber fibers. The amount of rubber will control the amount of tension that can be generated by the bandage. Even a bandage capable of generating moderate to strong tension still has so much elasticity that it can provide only minimal support. For this reason, elastic bandages should not be used to support an injured joint or muscle group.

When correctly applied, the elastic bandage is extremely useful for helping to control swelling in both chronic and acute injuries. Also, the elasticity of the bandage makes it ideal for securing protective pads and analgesic (balm) packs with little danger of causing muscle cramps due to the restriction of soft tissues.

The use of an elastic bandage as part of the RICE treatment of a new injury was discussed on page 64. After the initial treatment, mild support and control of swelling can be continued by applying a dry elastic bandage. This is more effective than tape strapping since the elastic bandage will "give" as tissues swell to help prevent a pressure buildup, which can interfere with circulation. Unlike tape, an elastic bandage can be loosened if it becomes too tight without losing compression.

Care must be taken to ensure that an elastic bandage is not applied too tightly or too loosely. For compression, start the bandage at the far end of the extremity (distal end), then wrap the bandage so that each succeeding layer overlaps the previous one by one-half its width. Angle the bandage up one side and then down the other to form a herringbone pattern that will help maintain fit (see Figure 19.1). Each overlap should be progressively looser. In this way, a pressure gradient is established that will help with the return of blood to the heart. Check with the athlete to make sure that the bandage is comfortable. If it is too tight, it must be loosened to prevent swelling in the extremity.

If the athlete is not going to participate in practice or an athletic event, the bandage can

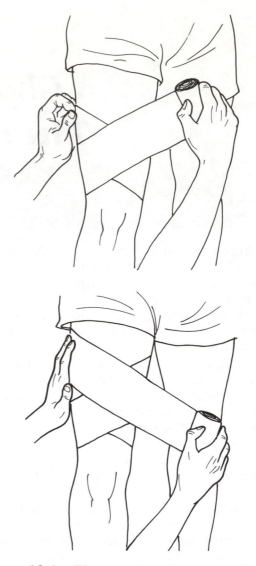

Figure 19.1. Wrap an elastic bandage with a one-half-width overlap to form a herringbone pattern.

be secured with the metal clips that are supplied with the bandage. Tape *must* be used to secure the bandage if the athlete is to participate. Clips and pins are too dangerous during participation.

Elastic bandages are available in 2-, 3-, 4-, and 6-inch widths. They may be purchased at most drug or sporting goods stores. There are double-length 4- and 6-inch bandages that are ideal for wrapping the thigh, but they may be difficult to locate for purchase. Another useful type of elastic bandage is the short 1½-inch size that can be used for the wrist.

All elastic bandages should be laundered in mild soap and warm water after each use. Hot water and strong detergents will cause the rubber to deteriorate. The same problem can occur due to hot-air drying. For this reason, it is best to air-dry the bandages. If this is not practical, place them in a dryer that is set for mild heat or air drying.

Ankle Wraps

These wraps are an inexpensive alternative to using tape strapping. The major advantage of these wraps is that cloth is reusable, but tape is not. You can use cotton twill that is 2 inches wide and cut in lengths varying from 72 to 96 inches. Your choice of an ankle-wrap pattern will determine which length is most efficient.

Most sporting goods stores and hospital supply companies can supply 38- or 72-yard lengths of ankle-wrap material. You also may be able to get some precut lengths from local sporting goods stores if only a few wraps are needed. The life of the wraps can be prolonged if you hem the ends. Each wrap must be laundered after use. Hot-air drying will not harm the material.

Athletic Tape

Since there are many different types and grades of athletic tape on the market, how can you decide which is the best buy for your needs? Here are some guidelines.

Quality

Higher grades of tape have more fibers woven per square inch than do the lower grades. They are stronger, but they are also more expensive. In addition to strength, you should consider the quality of the adhesive backing. It must be effective enough to keep the tape in place while the athlete is active and sweating. At the same time, the adhesive backing should not transfer to the athlete's skin and leave a residue. The adhesive should not transfer to the nonadhesive side of the tape (backcloth) when the tape is stored.

Porousness

Porous tape reduces the chances of skin irritation. It has tiny holes that are arranged systematically on the backing to permit air to pass through to the skin. Do not use waterproof tape. Waterproofing will make the tape less pliable.

Types of Tape

Athletic tape is available with a *serrated edge*, which is easy to tear, thus eliminating the need for scissors. Some tape has *zinc oxide* incorporated into the adhesive backing as an antiseptic to control skin irritation. This may prove to be a problem since some athletes have a sensitivity to the zinc oxide and will develop a skin irritation (contact dermatitis) when in contact with this type of tape.

Elastic tape is useful to solve taping problems caused by acute body angles. It can be used in combination with standard athletic tape. Use the elastic tape where you want a part to have more flexibility than is allowed by athletic tape; however, some support is lost to gain flexibility. For example, elastic tape is ideal for use as anchors in taping the knee because it allows the thigh muscles to contract and relax, thus reducing the chance of muscle cramping.

There are two types of elastic tape, one you can tear and one that must be cut with scissors. The size of elastic tape varies from 1 to 4 inches in width. The 1- inch width is for thumb taping and the 2- inch width for ankles and knees.

Clear plastic tape is often used for foot blisters since its use will reduce the friction created between the foot and shoe. It is perforated to allow air to circulate to the skin, which helps to reduce tissue damage that can occur due to the combined effects of friction and moisture.

Tension

The tension required to unroll the tape is important for the ease of application. Tape that unrolls smoothly without tugging or yanking will produce the most effective shaping and reduce wrinkles and stress on underlying tissues that may cause blister formation.

Size

The most efficient size of athletic tape is 1½-inch tape. Wider tape is rarely needed. You might need ½-inch wide tape for fingers and toes; however, the 1½-inch tape can be torn easily to produce these narrow strips.

Storing Tape Supplies

A tape storage area should be cool and dry to maintain optimum adhesiveness. Several rolls of tape can be placed in a refrigerator to help stabilize the adhesive. This tape must be warmed to room temperature before it is used. Be sure that the rolls of tape are stacked upright on their flat edges. A roll that has remained on one side for a period of time will become flattened and harder to unroll. More important than the difficulty you will experience in applying the tape is the uneven tension that will weaken the strapping and lead to blisters and tape burns.

If you have adequate storage space, you should consider buying tape by the case to reduce cost. You can calculate roughly what your needs for a season might be on the basis that you will need an average of a half of a roll per ankle. One case has enough tape to allow for the strapping of 64 ankles.

WORKING WITH TAPE

The trick to smooth tape application is to keep the roll close to the athlete's skin and the tape wound close to the roll (see Figure 19.2). This makes it easier to control both tension and placement. A slight bit of tension will allow the tape to conform to most body parts. Do not stretch the tape to make it conform as this will unduly stress the skin and increase the likelihood of irritation, tape burns, or cuts produced by the uneven pressure of the tape. The proper application of tape allows it to fall into place by guiding and molding it as you unroll the tape.

When using elastic tape, you will find it much more effective to unwind the tape a little further off the roll than you would with standard athletic tape. This reduces the tension. Too much stretching of elastic tape while strapping may restrict the athlete's circulation. A little practice is all that is necessary to develop the correct "feel" for the right amount of stretch required to apply elastic tape.

Taping will proceed more rapidly if you learn to tear the tape rather than stopping to cut it. To tear tape, you should follow these steps (see Figure 19.3):

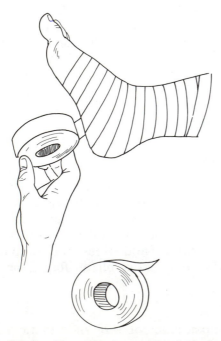

Figure 19.2. Keep the tape wound close to the roll and the roll close to the skin.

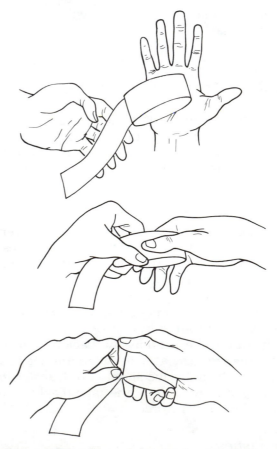

Figure 19.3. Procedures for tearing the tape with your fingers.

1. Hold the tape between the thumb and the index finger on each hand.
2. Place the thumbs close together.
3. Keep your wrists firm and push with one hand and pull with the other.
4. Tear with your fingers (not the fingernails), making certain that the edge of the tape is not bent over during the process.

You should learn to tape to an athlete's liking. Some athletes prefer to be taped tightly, while others can tolerate only a little pressure. Keep in mind that a loose strapping will irritate the skin and will offer virtually no support.

BASIC GUIDELINES

Taping is easier and more effective if you consider a few basic facts about the injury and the athlete. The seriousness of the injury and its degree of healing are important factors. Before taping, always ask yourself these questions:

- Should the injured athlete be practicing?
- Will participation aggravate the condition or predispose the athlete to reinjury or additional injuries?
- Will the injured athlete enjoy participating?

If you allow the injured athlete to return to activity, observe him or her closely. If it is evident that the injury affects performance, immediately take the athlete out of the event and treat the injury with the RICE method.

If the injury is less than 48-72 hours old, expect swelling. At this time, there is little reason to strap an injury for support or compression because the extent of the swelling is still unpredictable. If you tape the injury and it swells, increased pressure on the nerves and blood vessels may cause additional injury. Most athletes will, however, complain of discomfort and remove the tape before damage is done. A better approach is to apply an elastic bandage for compression and tell the athlete to loosen the bandage if it becomes too tight. If the athlete complains of numbness, tingling, or coldness or if you notice swelling below the bandage, the bandage *must* be loosened. Of course, this athlete should be restricted from

activity until the rehabilitation process has been completed.

Positioning of the Athlete

The position of the athlete while a body part is being taped will influence the effectiveness of the taping. For example, when strapping an ankle, have the athlete sit with the foot held at a relaxed right angle. When taping the knee, thigh, or groin, have the athlete stand. A 1-inch heel lift should be used when taping the knee. The athlete also should stand for the taping of an elbow, wrist, hand, or finger since it is easier to adjust the limb to a suitable height for strapping. A standing athlete is often more consciously involved in the strapping process and tends not to move the part as much. A good way to keep the wrist, hand, or thumb stabilized is to have the athlete place the fingers of the involved hand against the taper's abdomen. Taping is easier to accomplish if the athlete applies slight resistance against the pull of the tape as it is applied. A completely relaxed part has a tendency to move, and this will increase the chances of the tape being applied too tightly.

If you want to restrict joint movement, place the injured part in a position opposite the movement that is to be restricted. For example, if you want to avoid hyperextension of the elbow (straightening beyond 180°), the athlete should bend the elbow slightly and hold it in this position until the strapping is completed. Even the slightest movement from this position will decrease the effectiveness of the strapping.

Modifying Taping Techniques

You may have to modify taping techniques to adjust to the body size or the sex of the athlete. The massive body structure of larger athletes places more force on the joints. Therefore, wider tape and more layers may be necessary for proper support. The application of a groin wrap on a male athlete is more difficult. Female athletes present the problem of breast tissue interfering with certain strapping techniques. Also, the female body in general has less muscle bulk, smaller body parts, and more curvature to which tape must be conformed.

Closeness to Muscles, Nerves, and Blood Vessels

Keep in mind that when a muscle mass is being taped, the muscles must have room to contract and relax, or muscle cramps may develop. Elastic tape will allow for expansion, but take care to wrap without undue tension and only when the muscle is contracted.

Never encircle the muscle mass completely with standard athletic tape. For example, if you are taping an ankle, do not tape the belly of the lower-leg muscle. Instead, stop your taping before you reach the main part of the calf muscle.

When major nerves and blood vessels run close to the surface of the skin (as in the back of the knee and the front of the elbow), pad the sensitive area first to protect it against the pressure imposed by the tape. For correct padding, apply a lubricant and cover the area with a gauze pad or sponge before strapping.

Sensitivity and Skin Condition

Tape is rarely applied to the skin. Even though direct skin application will provide maximum support, it also will traumatize the area. The skin can be protected from tape irritation by covering it with several layers of underwrap prior to taping.

An athlete may be allergic to one or more of the ingredients used in strapping (tape adherent, underwrap, or tape). Most problems are with the adherent or the tape. If the athlete has some sort of reaction, try eliminating one item at a time to determine the cause. Remember, neither the adherent nor the underwrap is essential for support.

Skin irritation can be eliminated or reduced by using a gauze bandage under the tape. A conforming, self-adherent gauze bandage is ideal but more costly than a plain gauze bandage. If you use a plain gauze bandage, you must take a "tuck" each time the roll is wound around a part that tapers. It is easier to use cotton stockinette than a plain gauze bandage, but the cost is higher. Remember to secure the stockinette to the skin to provide a good taping base.

Applying Underwrap

There are certain preparatory steps that you should take to control the irritation that taping can cause. If there is hair on the skin, have the athlete shave the area to reduce the irritation to the hair follicles. Before applying the protective underwrap, spray the area with tape adherent and allow it to dry completely. The tape adherent will provide a tacky base for the tape and will reduce the growth of microorganisms.

To apply underwrap, keep it wound closely to the roll and have the roll kept close to the athlete's skin. Underwrap will become unmanageable if it is allowed to become unwound. If it rolls up, you must start again to help prevent blisters and discomfort. Stretch the underwrap slightly but not enough to cause it to roll up when applied. If the underwrap is applied at too acute an angle, it is also likely to roll up. It is best to let the underwrap fall in place naturally as you guide the roll. For example, in preparing an ankle for strapping, use a series of successive circular turns and a few figure eights to cover the heel and lace areas.

Always apply anchor strips of tape to the bottom and top edges of the underwrap, making them loose enough to avoid hampering circulation but not so loose that the underwrap is not held securely or there is a gap between the tape and the underwrap. If possible, start and end each strip of tape on the anchor, which will avoid unduly stressing the skin. If a strapping feels uncomfortable to the athlete, cut it off and redo the whole pattern. A strapping cannot be "broken in" and may interfere with nerve or circulatory function or cause tissue damage.

When taping an ankle, protect the heel and lace areas of the foot with gauze pads or sponges to prevent wear on these pivot points. Put a little lubricant on the pad to help cut down friction between the tape and the skin. Also, pad any bony areas, superficial tendons, and sensitive tissues (moles, wounds, and so on). Make certain that there are no openings or wrinkles in the underwrap, especially in the first layer as these may cause cuts and blisters.

Applying Tape

Do not use old tape or rolls with square edges. Improper storing can cause rolls to flatten. Such tape will cause unequal tension to be applied during the taping process. Pulling hard on the tape will serve only to put stress on the skin and underlying structures that may produce tape cuts, burns, and irritation to the hair follicles. This may lead to secondary infection and impairment of nerve and circulatory function.

As you begin to work with the tape, keep each layer as smooth as possible. Wrinkles in the tape will create areas of friction that will become sites of irritation. The first layer of tape is the critical one. Look carefully at the shape of the body part. If it tapers, you will have to angle the tape *upward* to conform to the contour. Work slowly to ensure a wrinkle-free application. If you have difficulty tearing tape, use precut lengths until you have mastered the skill.

Use an overlapping of one-third to one-half the width of the tape to provide maximum stability. If you allow the skin to gap through a separation between tape layers, a tape burn will probably occur.

A continuous strapping may have a tourniquet effect that will shut off blood flow. There is a tendency to pull the tape tightly to make it conform to the part. The tight tape places pressure on the blood vessels passing through the area and may interfere with blood flow. Using several segments of tape rather than one continuous piece of tape in strapping an injured body part is recommended.

Removing Tape

You should keep the time that the tape remains on the athlete to a minimum since

- the effectiveness of strapping decreases with time, and
- the chances of skin problems increase with time.

It is best to schedule taping sessions just prior to the practice or competition. Remember to leave sufficient time for a complete warm-up.

Remove all taping immediately following an activity. If more than one practice or event is scheduled during the same day, restrap the part before each activity period. Otherwise, the original taping will have lost its effectiveness and the moist environment and macerated skin under the tape provide an ideal situation for the development of bacterial or fungal infections. Remember that the chance of skin irrita-

tion is increased by the action of loose tape against moist skin.

The proper way to remove tape is by cutting through the layers of tape with a tape cutter (see Figure 19.4). Do *not* use bandage scissors as a general practice as their use increases the risk of injury and makes tape removal more difficult as the scissors become dull from cutting through multiple layers of tape. In some cases, a tape cutter may not be sufficient or available and bandage scissors will be necessary. In such situations, make certain that the scissors are sharp enough to do the job.

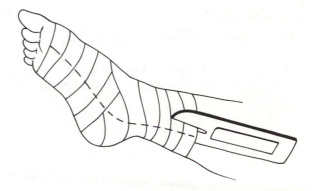

Figure 19.4. Using tape cutters to remove tape.

Always apply a little lubricant to the tip of the tape cutter to allow it to glide over the skin with little resistance and irritation. Once the strapping has been cut, use one hand to peel the tape away from the skin while using the other hand to push the skin away from the tape. *Do not yank the tape* as this only increases the likelihood of cuts and blisters.

If a tape-adhesive residue is left on the skin and is allowed to build up day after day, skin irritation will result. You should routinely remove the residue and tape adherent each time a tape job is removed. Commercial tape removers are available at most sporting goods stores. Oil-based fingernail polish remover also works, but it is expensive and may irritate some athletes' skin. Whenever a tape remover is used, be certain to wash the skin thoroughly with soap and water to reduce the chances of irritation.

EFFECTIVENESS OF TAPING

Taping is effective if the athlete has confidence in it because it looks good and is comfortable, if it accomplishes its intended purposes, and if it holds up to the stress of the activity. It takes time and practice to acquire taping skills. Forget about speed and concentrate on the proper placement of the strips and on neatness. In the next chapter some specific taping patterns will be discussed. You should practice each technique several times before attempting to tape a rehabilitating athlete. Once you feel confident in your taping abilities, then you may use the techniques. Apply taping techniques *only* when an athlete has received medical consent to return to full activity.

SUMMARY AND RECOMMENDATIONS

Taping is part of a good rehabilitation program, but it does *not* replace the rehabilitation program! New injuries should not be taped. Rather, taping should be used during the last part of rehabilitation to limit range of motion and to support healing tissues.

1. Proper taping requires you to consider the anatomy of the injured area and the movement and stress the area will undergo.
2. Most taping procedures require some sort of modification to better suit each individual athlete and to account for his or her specific injury.
3. Guidelines for selection of taping materials and methods to ensure adequate strapping were presented.

Chapter 20
Taping Patterns

The taping patterns detailed in this chapter are meant to be used at the final stage of rehabilitation. Do not attempt to simply read through this chapter. Instead, it is suggested that you study and practice each pattern before moving on to the next one.

All tape should be removed using tape cutters or bandage scissors. Household scissors are too dangerous to use.

LOWER-EXTREMITY TAPING

Special care must be taken when taping the lower extremities. The muscle masses, multiple joints, acute angles involved, and the forces that may be applied to the joints make effective therapeutic taping difficult enough to merit additional practice.

Taping the Ankle

Flexibility and support are required in the taping of the ankle. Take care not to give up one in favor of the other. If you find that flexibility must be reduced to give the needed support, then you must question whether the athlete is ready for the activity.

The Ankle Wrap

The materials required for the ankle wrap include 72 inches of cotton twill ankle wrap, 1½-inch athletic tape, and nonsterile gauze sponges (or "bubbles"). The athlete should hold the foot at a right angle throughout the wrapping process. Be certain that you pull the sock tight so the area to be wrapped is wrinkle free to avoid possible blistering.

The steps for wrapping the ankle include the following (see Figure 20.1):

1. Place a gauze sponge or bubbles over the lace and heel areas to pad the underlying tendons.
2. Because most ankle injuries result in pain or injury to the outside of the ankle, you want to restrict the turning in of the ankle. Start the wrap on the inside of the lower leg, directly over the top of the lace pad. Be sure to maintain a constant tension on the twill as you wrap the ankle. Ask the athlete if he or she prefers a tight or a loose wrap.
3. Keeping the correct tension, loop the wrap around the leg, over the heel pad, and across the top of the foot to the middle of the inner arch.
4. Bring the wrap under the foot and over the top of the heel pad. The wrap should be pulled upward so that it goes on a diagonal, across the outside of the heel. This is referred to as a *heel lock*.
5. Continue to pull the wrap around the heel to the inside of the leg.
6. Bring the wrap around the ankle to serve as an anchor point.
7. Angle the wrap across the top of the foot to the middle of the outer arch.
8. Pull the wrap under the foot and angle it upward so that it catches the inside of the heel on a diagonal. This is a *heel lock*.
9. Continue by carrying the wrap up behind the heel to the outside of the leg.
10. Bring the wrap around the ankle to finish off the heel lock.
11. Now, start a figure eight by drawing the wrap down across the top of the foot to the middle of the inner arch.
12. Pull the wrap under the foot to the middle of the outer arch.
13. Angle the wrap across the top of the foot.

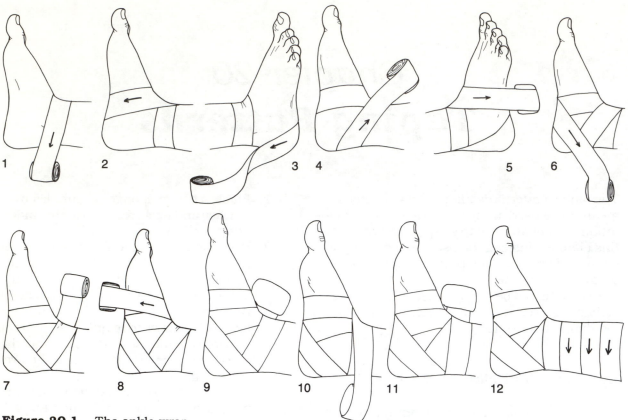

Figure 20.1. The ankle wrap.

14. Loop the wrap around the lower leg from the inside to the outside just above the ankle. This finishes the pattern. If any wrap is left over, continue to loop it around the lower leg. Each successive layer should overlap the previous one by one-half its width.

15. Anchor the end of the strip with tape. For added support, retrace the figure eight (Steps 12-15) with tape.

Ankle Strapping (Closed Basketweave)

The materials needed for ankle strapping include tape adherent, underwrap, 1½-inch athletic tape, gauze sponges ("bubbles"), and lubricant. Instruct the athlete to hold the foot at a right angle throughout the strapping process.

Before taping can begin, the ankle must be prepared. Spray or paint the entire area with tape adherent and allow it to dry. Next, apply a lubricant to two protective pads. Place one pad at the "lace" area and the other at the heel to protect the underlying tendons. Finally, use underwrap to cover the entire area from the ball of the foot to the lower border of the belly of the calf muscle (gastrocnemius).

The steps for taping an inversion sprain (sole turned inward) of the ankle are as follows (see Figure 20.2):

1. Apply the first anchor strip loosely around the sole of the foot. The tape need not be in contact with the skin to secure the underwrap. Initially you will be more successful if you secure the underwrap to the skin. Remember, the foot will flatten out as it bears the body's weight. Always leave the toes and joints clear.

2. Apply the second anchor strip around the shin, just below the belly of the calf muscle. You should angle the tape ends upward to conform to the taper of the leg. Usually, the tape does have to be in contact with the skin to secure the underwrap.

3. Place the first stirrup. Start on the inside of the leg at the anchor strip and bring the tape down the inside of the leg behind the anklebone (malleolus) and

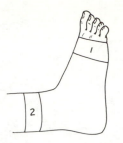
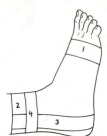
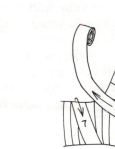
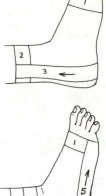
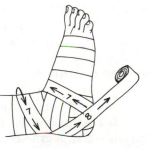

Figure 20.2.   The closed basketweave.

up the outside of the leg behind the anklebone. End on the anchor strip.

4. Apply the third anchor strip on the shin. Overlap the initial shin anchor by one-third to one-half its width. Angle the tape ends upward.

5. Lay down the first horseshoe. Start on the heel as close to the sole of the foot as possible. Pull the ends of the tape forward toward the toes and slightly downward toward the sole of the foot. End the tape on the anchor. If the tape is angled downward, it will conform to the taper of the heel. There should not

be an air bubble between the tape and underwrap at the heel.

6. Complete the stirrup, anchor, horseshoe pattern two more times. Make certain that

    • the tape overlaps the previous piece by one-third to one-half its width;

    • the second stirrup covers most of the ankle bone, and the third stirrup covers the rest of it;

    • the stirrups are kept within the heel area to avoid stress on the arch;

    • the shin anchors angle upward;

    • all horseshoes start on the heel with the tape ends angling slightly downward toward the sole of the foot. By making each succeeding horseshoe shorter than the previous one, a stair-step effect is created that will leave the shoelace area free of tape. Too much tape in this area will limit the athlete's range of motion.

7. Fill in the lower leg with anchor strips. Angle the tape ends slightly upward, overlapping one-third to one-half. They should crisscross on the front of the lower leg.

8. Fill in the arch, applying the tape loosely around the foot.

9. Create a figure eight with tape. Start on the inside of the leg with the roll of tape. Fix the end of the tape just below the anklebone and loop the roll around the back of the leg and across the top of the foot. Encircle the arch and end on top of the foot. The tape should cross the middle of the inner and outer arches.

10. Secure the first heel lock. Start on the inside of the leg at the top anchor strip and angle the tape downward across the front of the shin. Try to keep the tape at a 45° angle as it reaches the ankle. Loop the tape around the back of the leg, just above the heel (over the top of the Achilles tendon). It will be necessary to angle the tape downward to catch the inside edge of the heel. Continue the taping so that it goes diagonally across the bottom of the foot to end on the inside surface of the leg.

11. Secure the second heel lock. Follow the same pattern used for the first heel lock but start on the outside of the leg, catching the outside edge of the heel.

12. Apply lock strips. Start on the leg, just below the belly of the calf muscle. Overlap the strips by one-third to one-half.

Taping Shin Splints

When taping of the lower leg is done too tightly, severe restrictions are placed on the muscles of the lower leg. Additional care must be exercised to avoid any taping pattern that will greatly restrict action at the knee or the ankle. Never completely encircle a muscle mass with nonelastic tape.

Most attending physicians with background in sports medicine will recommend arch taping for athletes with shin splints because the inflamed muscles provide primary muscular support for the arches. The materials required for arch taping include tape adherent, 1- and/or 1½-inch athletic tape, and underwrap. Instruct the athlete to hold the foot at a right angle throughout the entire procedure.

The athlete should sit with his or her injured leg extended and the foot held at a right angle. Prior to taping, spray or paint the area with tape adherent. Allow this to dry and then cover the foot with underwrap.

The procedure for taping arches is as follows (see Figure 20.3):

1. Apply an anchor strip loosely around the foot (the foot will spread out as weight is borne). The strip need not come in contact with the skin.
2. Start at the anchor on the sole of the foot. Angle the tape from the lateral (little-toe) side of the foot, across the sole, around the heel, and along the outside of the foot as close to the sole as possible. End on the anchor strip.
3. Repeat this process at the anchor on the sole of the foot, but this time begin on the medial (big-toe) side. Angle the tape across the sole, around the heel, and along the inside of the foot as close to the sole as possible. End on the anchor strip. *Note:* If you are using 1-inch tape, repeat steps 2 and 3.
4. Apply two or three locking strips loosely around the foot, allowing for the foot to spread when weight is borne. Overlap the strips by one-third to one-half.
5. If necessary, apply arch pads.

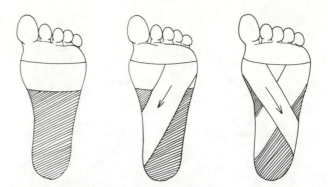

Figure 20.3. Taping arches.

Taping the front of the shin is of limited use in rehabilitation but does offer a little extra support and may help relieve some pain and fatigue. The materials required for this procedure include tape adherent, 1½-inch athletic tape, and elastic wrap. During the application of the tape and wrap, the athlete should be seated on a table, with the knee bent and the foot held flat on the table surface. Before beginning to tape, spray or paint the area of the lower leg with tape adherent.

The taping procedure for the front of the shin is as follows:

1. Tape the arch first.
2. Place two vertical anchor strips, one on each side of the leg. Each strip should begin just above the ankle and end just above the belly of the calf.
3. Apply short strips of tape across the shin. Each strip should be applied at a slightly upward angle and secured to each anchor strip. Begin at the ankle and work upward in a crisscrossed fashion (see Figure 20.4).
4. The short strips of tape are held in place by vertical strips placed over the anchor strips.
5. At the option of the attending physician, elastic wrap may be applied around the shin. This is usually discontinued as rehabilitation nears completion.

Wrapping the Thigh

Wrapping can be done to offer support for the anterior muscle mass of the thigh (the quadriceps). This is usually done for pulls and severe bruising. Tape adherent, 1½- or 2-inch tape, and 3-inch elastic tape or one 6-inch elastic

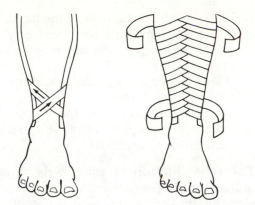

Figure 20.4. Taping the front of the shin.

bandage will be required. Taping for support requires you to do the following:

1. Prepare the site and apply tape adherent.
2. Apply one long vertical anchor strip each along the inside and outside of the front of the thigh. Fold the tape in half lengthwise so there is adhesive to stick to both the leg and the elastic wrap if you are using the 6-inch elastic bandage.
3. Starting about 2 inches above the knee, apply strips of tape so that they overlap and cross one another to create an X pattern (see Figure 20.5). The strips must start at the bottom of one anchor strip and end toward the top of the other.
4. Apply locking strips of tape along the same lines as the anchor strips.
5. Continue making Xs across the front of the thigh by overlapping the strips of each previous X by one-half the width of the tape. Stop when you have covered the front of the thigh.
6. Some physicians will want added support provided by having you bandage the thigh with elastic tape or bandage, while others will not wish to have this much restriction applied.

The same technique is used to support the hamstrings as was employed to support the quadriceps except that the X pattern is created over the back of the thigh.

THE UPPER EXTREMITIES

Therapeutic taping of the upper extremities is usually associated with the rehabilitation of

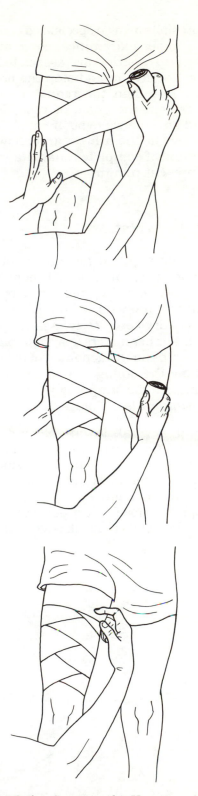

Figure 20.5. Creating the X pattern in wrapping the thigh.

strains, minor sprains, and other mild injuries. The procedures are typically done to limit the motion of a specific joint in all directions. Since many sport skills involve specialized conditioning of the upper extremities, some athletes may object to restrictions associated with taping. Do not give in and stop the program or provide less than the required support. Instead, explain the goals of rehabilitation taping and how the way you are applying the tape will benefit the athlete and allow for a shorter period of complete rehabilitation and possibly prevent reinjury.

Taping the Wrist

The materials required for taping the wrist include tape adherent, 1½- or 1-inch athletic tape, and underwrap. Prepare the area by spraying or painting the wrist with tape adherent. Allow this to dry completely. Ask the athlete to spread his or her fingers apart and place his or her fingertips on the abdomen of the person who is doing the taping.

Following are the strapping procedures for *minimal support* (see Figure 20.6):

1. Wrap several layers of underwrap around the wrist. This band should be approximately 2 inches wide and should extend beyond the wrist to the base of the hand.
2. Apply a strip of tape around the far end of the wrist so that the edge of the tape

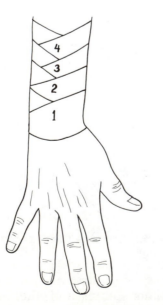

Figure 20.6. Taping the wrist for minimal support.

overlaps onto the base of the hand. The tape will conform more easily if you angle the tape ends down toward the hand. Do *not* pull the tape too tight. Also, make certain that the fingers remain spread apart.

3. Repeat the circular strips two or three times, overlapping the previous strip by one-third to one-half.

The rehabilitation of some wrist injuries requires limiting wrist flexion or extension. Following are the taping procedures offering *moderate support* (see Figure 20.7).

1. Wrap several layers of underwrap around the palm and wrist in a figure-eight pattern. Apply one or two layers of underwrap at the wrist and then angle up across the back of the hand, between the thumb and index finger, and down across the palm. Repeat this process twice.
2. Place an anchor strip around the forearm, about 3 inches above the wrist (styloid processes).
3. Place a second anchor strip just below the knuckles, keeping the fingers spread during the process.
4. The wrist must be moved (flexed or extended) in the direction opposite that which causes discomfort and kept in this position until the procedure is completed.
5. Use strips of tape to form a crisscross pattern. To restrict flexion of the wrist, apply tape to the back of the hand; to restrict extension, apply tape to the palm. Begin the first strip at the anchor below the little finger, pull it across the wrist, and attach it to the forearm anchor. The second strip is applied to the anchor below the index finger. Pull it across the wrist and attach it to the forearm anchor. This crisscross pattern is repeated three more times.
6. Two figure-eight patterns of taping are applied over the top of the crisscross pattern.

Taping the Palm

This method is used to protect healed rips in the palm of the hand and may be useful in pre-

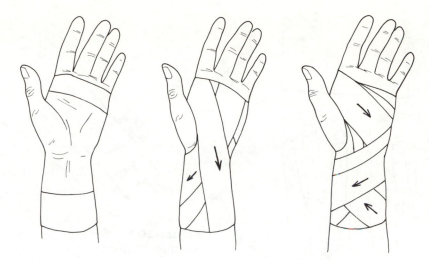

Figure 20.7.   Taping the wrist for moderate support of extension injury.

venting rips often associated with gymnastics. Do *not* use this procedure on freshly opened rips even if sealants and first aid creams are available as this may contaminate the wound.

Do *not* have the athlete participate if any rips to the palm are not healed. Simple taping may not prevent additional damage. The exception is the athlete with successful but incomplete healing of a rip who is granted a physician's approval to participate. In such cases, ask the physician if you can paint the wound site with a flexible collodion (e.g., New Skin) to seal the wound. If this is not possible, apply a gauze pad with first aid cream.

The materials needed for rip taping include tape adherent, 1½-inch athletic tape, and 2- or 3-inch plastic tape. Paint or spray the palm and wrist with tape adherent and allow it to dry before taping. Keep the athlete's fingers spread during the entire taping process.

Rip taping requires the following steps (see Figure 20.8):

1. Apply underwrap and secure it with an anchor strip of 1½-inch athletic tape around the wrist.
2. Cut a piece of elastic tape so that it is long enough to cover both the front and the back of the hand when the tape is stretched.
3. Fold the elastic tape's nonsticky sides together and cut two small triangles out of the folded edge.
4. Slip the third and fourth fingers of the athlete's hand through the triangles and pull the elastic tape along the back of the hand so that the edges of the tri-

angles are as close to the fingers as possible. This will provide more protection for the palm.
5. End the elastic tape on the back of the hand at the wrist anchor.
6. Cup the athlete's hand slightly and stretch the elastic tape across the palm, ending it on the wrist anchor.
7. Secure the elastic tape ends by applying a strip of 1½-inch athletic tape around the wrist. Make sure that the athlete has the fingers spread.

Leather handgrips may be worn over the top of the tape grips for additional protection; however, some athletes find that using both forms of protection is too bulky and often causes them to lose their grip.

Taping the Fingers

The materials needed for finger taping include tape adherent, 1- or ½-inch athletic tape, and gauze sponges or pads. To prepare for taping, you should spray or paint the injured finger and an adjoining uninjured finger with tape adherent. An injured ring finger should be secured to the little finger, leaving the middle and index fingers free. In the taping procedure, always try to leave the index finger free. Next, cut a strip of gauze wide enough and long enough to fit between the two fingers. Tear two to four strips of tape so that they are long enough to circle both fingers and overlap slightly.

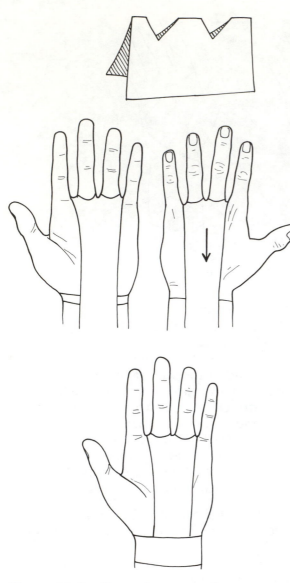

Figure 20.8.   Using elastic tape for taping "rips."

The remaining procedures for finger taping include the following (see Figure 20.9):

1. Place the gauze strip between the two fingers so that it will serve as a pad.
2. Wrap one strip of tape around the base of the fingers, leaving the joints free. You may need to split the tape lengthwise for a narrower width. The joints *must* be able to flex so that they can give when a force is applied.
3. Apply a second strip of tape around the fingers between the second and third joints.
4. Repeat Steps 2 and 3 if additional reinforcement is needed.

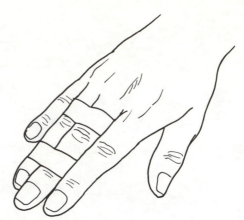

Figure 20.9.   Secure the injured finger to an uninjured finger.

Taping the Thumb

Most often, any therapeutic taping of the thumb is done as part of the rehabilitation of a minor thumb sprain. The materials needed include tape adherent and 1-inch athletic tape. The procedure requires you to do the following (see Figure 20.10):

1. Apply tape adherent around the wrist and base of the thumb.
2. Place one anchor strip around the wrist. Keep this anchor loose.
3. Place another anchor at the distal end of the thumb.
4. Four strips of tape should be applied from anchor to anchor along the injured side of the thumb (back or palm side). These should be held in place with one strip of tape applied around the wrist and a second strip placed around the distal thumb.
5. Three additional strips of tape (spica) are added. When pain occurs with movement away from the midline (abduction), start the first strip at the base of the thumb on the palm side of the hand. Angle this strip upward under the thumb, encircle it, and bring the tape around to the back (dorsal side) of the hand. The tape should crisscross over the outside of the thumb to form an X. Fold over the edge of the tape as you apply it to the web space to reduce irritation. Continue the tape around the wrist and end at the starting point to form a figure eight. Place the second

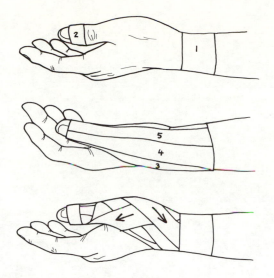

Figure 20.10. Taping the thumb to restrict movement away from the midline (abduction).

strip so that it will overlap the first one by two-thirds, and encircle the thumb at a more distal point. The third strip should be applied the same way, overlapping the second strip by two-thirds. Be careful not to encircle the thumb too tightly; circulation can easily be hindered.

6. Apply an anchor strip at the wrist to secure the tape ends.

This method of thumb taping will help protect the joints and muscles of the thumb, especially in cases involving pain during abduction (away from the midline). If the pain occurs on adduction (movement toward the midline), the same basic procedure is applied; however, the spicas are applied starting at the base of the thumb on the dorsal surface.

SUMMARY AND RECOMMENDATIONS

Tape for rehabilitation is not meant to be applied so that the athlete can have additional support to rejoin the activity before proper healing has taken place.

1. Taping is meant to be part of a physician-approved program.
2. The proper application of each taping technique requires practicing the specific technique and modifications to allow the taping to fit the athlete.

References

DeLorme, T. L., & Watkins, W. L. (1955). *Progressive resistance exercise.* New York: Appleton-Century-Crofts.

Nygaard, G., & Boone, T. H. (1985). *Coaches guide to sport law.* Champaign, IL: Human Kinetics.

Sharkey, B.J. (1986). *Coaches guide to sport physiology.* Champaign, IL: Human Kinetics.

Index

(*cont.*)